DIABETES:

A Guide to Living Well

A Program
of Individualized Self-Care

**Ernest Lowe
and Gary Arsham, M.D., Ph.D.**

Foreword by Peter Forsham, M.D.

Diabetes: A Guide to Living Well © 1992 by Ernest Lowe and Gary
Arsham, M.D.

Library of Congress Cataloging-in-Publication Data

Arsham, Gary M.
      Diabetes: a guide to living well.
      Includes bibliographical references and index
      ISBN 0-937721-51-4
      1. Diabetes—Popular works. I. Lowe, Ernest. II. Title.
      RC660.4.A77 1992   616.4'62   88-31040
                                   CIP

Cover and text design: Terry Dugan Design
Editor: Donna Hoel
Typesetting: Wordex, Lory Strom

Published by
CHRONIMED Publishing
P.O. Box 47945
Minneapolis, MN 55447-9727

Table of Contents

SECTION V: LIVING WELL WITH DIABETIC COMPLICATIONS

Dedication

To Diana Silver Arsham and Grace O'Rielly Lowe who could easily write a sequel to this book called **Diabetics: A Guide to Living Well With Them.**

To my parents, Florence and Sanford Arsham and my physician while growing up, Max Miller, who gave me the guidance and freedom to live well. — *Gary*

To John Menscher and Michael Barricks, whose skilled laser treatment enabled me to keep 20/20 vision. — *Ernest*

Acknowledgments

Many people have made valuable contributions to **Diabetes: A Guide to Living Well**—fellow diabetics (patients and friends) and professional colleagues.

We wish to thank Everett Ai, Carol Alston, Robert Barnes, Peter Barrett, Patrick Bean, Ken Burke, Philip R. Calanchini, Larry Catus, Cathy Corum, Leona Dang, Wayne Davis, Joan Enns, Fran Fernandez, Betty Fukuyama, Diana Guthrie, Dwight Holing, Peggy Huang, Larry Hulbert, Chris Kilduff, Barry S. Levin, Maureen McGrath, Fran Nereu, Jan Norman, Linda Parker, Sheila Perez, Donna Radcliffe, Vicky Sears, Nanci Stern, Wendy Ullman-Duarte, Helen Wall, Ben and Bonnie Weyhing, Seena Wolf, patients of the Early Treatment Diabetic Retinopathy Study, and the many others who supported our work with their knowledge and experience.

Special thanks go to George Cleveland, formerly of Diabetes Center, Inc., and Caroline Danielson, our editor for the first edition, for helping to bring this book to completion. We are grateful to Donna Hoel and David Wexler of DCI/CHRONIMED for their assistance and guidance with the second edition.

Foreword

by Peter Forsham, M.D., Professor of Medicine and Pediatrics, Emeritus, and former Director, Metabolic Research Unit, University of California, San Francisco. (Dr. Forsham has had diabetes for 68 years.)

Diabetes: A Guide to Living Well is one of the few books to acknowledge a difficult fact of life. There are three kinds of diabetics: those who cooperate completely in maintaining a normal blood glucose range; those who do this part time; and those who never do it. The authors, all type I diabetics for many years, provide guidance appropriate to all three groups.

This book covers all the modern ways of maintaining a normal blood sugar level (not usually exceeding 130 mg;dl) and introduces in a philosophical way the persuasive reasons for doing this. At the same time, the authors support the individual's right to choose his or her level of self-care, and they recognize that many choose a level far below the standard now attainable. Their unique contribution is to offer alternative strategies for increasing the reader's willingness to follow regimens valuable in diabetes management. Throughout, the hope is expressed that through lifelong learning and adequate teaching by his or her medical team, the reader will become increasingly wise.

The authors write from a powerful combination of personal and professional experience. Not only have they lived with diabetes for many years, but they've also surveyed advanced research in diabetes and medical education to uncover the most effective techniques for improving self-care and adherence to reasonable regimens. They dismiss ignorant old beliefs, some harking back to the days before insulin, when diabetics were absolutely forbidden sugar and were told to stay in a mild state of ketoacidosis to survive. Unfortunately, such misinformation from the past still fills some diabetes texts. This book makes little of the old prejudices, introducing instead the latest concepts in treatment of diabetes.

Beginning with tips on mastering the challenge of learning a complex regimen, the book is an operating manual for the individual who wishes to maintain the best possible level of diabetic control. It wisely charts alternative paths for those prepared to quickly gain this goal and those who prefer to move more gradually.

The authors accept the concept that hyperglycemia (or high blood sugar levels) is what I once called toxic. Today we know that the prevention of general vascular disease in diabetics is a function of the control of blood glucose, cholesterol, and fat levels in the blood. This is an essential component in the reduction of the risk of diabetic complications involving the eyes, kidneys, nerves, and circulatory system. This Guide to Living Well imparts knowledge enabling the reader to manage fat intake on the one hand and to prevent hyperglycemia on the other.

The crowning achievement of this book, however, is its full synthesis of all factors affecting blood sugar level. On the deficit side, mental instability, stress, lack of exercise or rest, and dietary excess, each through different mechanisms, raise the blood sugar level and accelerate the degenerative processes of diabetes. But when a diabetic assumes a regimen integrating mental balance, stress management, dietary moderation, and exercise, he or she is reducing long-term risks and ensuring more immediate well-being.

The authors realistically offer routes to this ideal of self-management suited to a broad range of personalities, not just those immediately capable of strong discipline.

In the 1860s, Claude Bernard observed that the condition for a free existence is the constancy of the internal environment. Now people with diabetes can hope to approach this metabolic constancy by controlling the multiple factors that are abnormal in the average patient. This aim is deeply supported by this very practical yet highly philosophical newcomer to the diabetes information scene.

Preface

We wrote **Diabetes: A Guide to Living Well** to give you (1) a command of one of medicine's most demanding regimens; (2) mastery over the threats diabetes presents; and (3) strength to meet its emotional challenges. Throughout the book, we encourage you to choose a regimen individualized to your personal needs and preferences. Most important, we present strategies empowering you to follow the regimen you choose. We wrote this book so you can learn to live well with diabetes.

The **Living Well** approach is based on the dual experience each of us brings to the book. We know diabetes professionally and personally. (Your writing team has logged a total of 182 years of living with diabetes!) We temper medical experts' views with first-hand knowledge of the challenges, threats, and gifts of diabetes.

The basic diabetes lifestyle is a thorough program with a strong unity. Control of blood sugar levels is important in avoiding short-term crises, in maintaining a feeling of well-being, and in reducing your risk of long-term diabetic complications. Blood sugar control, along with an active life, balanced diet, and effective stress management, work together to reduce your risk of complications. Emotional balance and self-esteem contribute to stress management and aid you in following your self-care program. Remembering this unity is central to the **Living Well** approach.

While we devote many pages to the question of blood glucose control, we emphasize throughout the book that you live well by balancing metabolic control with all other aspects of your lifestyle. When you do this, you integrate diabetes into your life and keep it from dominating you.

Individual choice is central to the **Living Well** approach and can easily be applied while using this book. It is not necessarily a book to be read from front to back. You know better than anyone else what you need to learn first. We encourage you to follow your own sense of priorities.

You may have much to learn, many skills to gain, and behaviors to change as you adopt the **Living Well** approach, especially if you are new to diabetes. Throughout this book, you will find ideas for making this process of learning and changing easier to handle. You will also find many techniques for increasing your willingness to follow this life-enhancing and demanding self-care regimen.

Ingredients of the Living Well With Diabetes Lifestyle

Find a balance between meeting your needs as a diabetic and the other needs in your life. Chapters 1 and 4 offer guidance on striking this balance.

- Know how to avoid the acute, life-threatening crises of diabetes. We have highlighted basic life-saving guidelines at the back of this book. Chapter 8 contains a thorough discussion of insulin reactions.

- Know the measures you can take to reduce the risk of developing diabetic complications. Preventive measures are discussed in Chapter 15 and 17.

- Maintain the best control of blood glucose levels you can achieve without damaging the quality of your life. Chapters 4 through 7 offer a choice of regimens and instructions for each.

- Meet your emotional needs, not just your physical needs. Chapter 14 presents a variety of techniques for maintaining emotional well-being. Chapter 3 describes techniques for dealing with crisis.

- Manage stress effectively. Chapter 11 describes the impact of stress on diabetes and techniques for coping with it.

- Maintain an active lifestyle, adjusted to your physical condition. Chapter 10 explores the role of exercise in diabetes management.

- Follow a balanced and moderate diet. Chapter 9 gives tips on making your diet delicious as well as healthy.

- Work to increase your willingness to follow this lifestyle, and continue learning about it. Chapter 1 surveys actions and beliefs that support continuing adherence to the self-care program you choose. Chapter 3 includes techniques to help you handle the times when you want to rebel.

A fundamental guideline to using this book

Diabetes is a condition requiring a balance between your own day-to-day decision making in self-care and your doctor's guidance on basic regimen decisions. We include detailed information on three regimens so you can work with your physician in making decisions about insulin dosage; overall balance between insulin, diet, and exercise; or treatment of acute crises like ketoacidosis. In no way do we encourage you to make these fundamental medical decisions on your own.

In writing this book, we have deepened our own capacity for living well with diabetes. We hope reading it helps you do the same.

Gary Arsham

Ernest Lowe

TO THE PHYSICIAN AND OTHER HEALTH CARE TEAM MEMBERS

Diabetes: A Guide to Living Well is intended to help your patient to not only live well with diabetes, but also to be a better, more informed, more responsible patient. As you know, with a chronic illness like diabetes, what patients do outside your office is critical to their medical care. You can recommend, monitor, guide, encourage, and exhort, but it is your patient who does or does not follow what the two of you agree is an appropriate regimen.

This book provides considerable information that should make your patient much more informed and motivated to work with you and other members of the health care team. It encourages the patient to examine the options available, consider the risks and benefits as we understand them today, and, in collaboration with you, choose a level of diabetes management and control that fits the individual situation. We hope this book will help your patient and also make your tasks more satisfying and rewarding.

TO INCREASE YOUR CHANCES FOR A LONGER, MORE HEALTHFUL LIFE

Living well with diabetes means preserving your health and vitality and reducing your risk of developing future diabetic complications. Improving blood sugar control is just one of the things you can do to achieve these goals. The complete Living Well lifestyle asks you to

- Improve your control of blood glucose and continue improving it to the best level you are comfortable with (Chapters 4-7).

- Learn to handle stress well (Chapter 11).

- Follow a diabetic diet that features low animal fat and high fiber as well as limited sweets and rapidly absorbed carbohydrates (Chapter 9).

- Exercise regularly (Chapter 10).

- Lose weight if you are overweight.

- Act to prevent high blood pressure by controlling stress, weight, and salt consumption. Seek treatment for hypertension if your blood pressure is high (above 140/90) (Chapter 17, hypertension section).

- Get the amount of sleep and rest you need.

- Know the warning signs for each complication. Begin treatment early if symptoms appear (Chapter 17).

- Consider taking a multivitamin pill daily.

These preventive measures are discussed in detail in Chapter 17. You should also skim through that chapter to find the sections describing what you can do to prevent individual complications.

A note on style: Although the noun diabetic has become controversial, we have chosen to use it in *Living Well*. We find nothing negative in the word itself. Being a diabetic is but one of the many roles we fill in life. Naming that role when it is appropriate does not make that our sole identity.

Section I
LEARNING TO LIVE WELL

Introduction

"Nobody asked me if I wanted to have diabetes. I just started feeling lousy, losing weight, and getting thirsty. And there I was—diabetic. I thought my life was ruined. But then I said, 'No, dammit! This may not go away, but I'm going to call the shots. My life is more than a defective pancreas.'"

— John, 45 years old, twenty-five years diabetic

"The anger, the frustration, and all of these feelings aren't going to take the diabetes away. You have to find a level ground and decide, 'Okay, this is the way I am now and I'd better learn what I'm supposed to do and what I'm not supposed to do and live with it, because that's the way it's going to be.'"

— Norma, 58 years old
(In *Focus on Feelings,* from Pyramid Films)

We can choose how to live with diabetes. We can't decide not to have it, but we can decide to live a full and satisfying life, rejecting all images of ourselves as ill or disabled. No matter what your physical condition is, we can choose to live well. The act of choosing becomes the foundation of our ability to manage diabetes effectively.

Living well depends less on how we care for our diabetes than on how we care for ourselves. Each of us has a whole pattern of living that includes our individual needs, style, abilities, and physical characteristics. The diabetic regimen we choose will work only if it fits with this pattern. We cannot make decisions about diabetes care as if diabetes is the only thing we have to consider in life.

For this reason, the authors of *Diabetes: A Guide to Living Well* — insulin-dependent diabetics themselves—emphasize your right to select a self-care program, in conjunction with your physician and health care team, that will work for you as an individual. We encourage you to read this book in whatever order feels right to you. Work on the subjects that appeal to you the most. Find the level of regimen you believe you can follow comfortably. Work to find the right balance between quality of life and care of diabetes. When you exercise this freedom of choice, you are likely to arrive at a program you can live with.

Throughout this book, we have interwoven advice on how you can build willingness to follow the regimen you choose with information on the physical and emotional care of diabetes. In the last decade, dramatic improvements have been made in diabetes care, changes that have made the state-of-the-art regimen more complex. Taking full advantage of these breakthroughs may require you to pay attention to the feelings, beliefs, and patterns of behavior that sometimes divide your will.

Living well with diabetes is easier if you are willing to continually learn about the rapidly changing field of diabetes control. There are many new skills to be gained and, often, behaviors need changing as information is updated. We have included hints and strategies in the book to make the learning process easier.

WHICH REGIMEN?

If you elect anything less than the strictest regimen, you may feel guilt, anxiety, or conflict for making a "bad" choice. On the one hand, these feelings are important to consider in your decision-making process. You must accept your level of care, or the quality of your life will suffer from the conflict you feel. However, to live well with diabetes, once you understand the risks and benefits of the different options and have made an informed choice, you must shed all feelings of conflict. Accept your decision. Realize that it is the best one for you.

Of course, we want to be certain that what we do to take care of ourselves will actually work. But the only certainty we can gain at this point is statistical: Excellent diabetic control reduces the risk of complications. A large percentage of us who maintain good control will escape blindness, kidney disease, nerve damage, and so on. But any one of us may do everything possible to control our diabetes and still experience some degree of disability because of the disease.

So, living well with diabetes calls for accepting uncertainty and staying motivated in the face of it. This is such a central issue that we ask you to explore your reactions to it in this questionnaire.

QUESTIONNAIRE: A CERTAIN UNCERTAINTY

1. As you read the last three paragraphs, how did you feel?

2. How do you handle uncertainties in areas of your life outside diabetes?

3. What attitudes or beliefs could you adopt that would help you deal with the uncertainties about your future that diabetes imposes?

4. What do you think would help motivate you to follow your diabetes management program, even though you have no guarantee that the program will prevent complications?

There are no simple formulas for handling these basic questions. Yet it is dangerous to avoid them. Negative reactions to uncertainty range from abandoning all efforts to manage diabetes to caring for it so compulsively that life holds little joy. Clearly, managing diabetes is a matter of balance—doing the best you can and then living as fully as you can, without dwelling on possible future misfortunes.

One way of neutralizing uncertainty about the future is to make the present moment rewarding. Learn to accept each moment as a source of benefit, no matter what happens. Then you are prepared for whatever the future may bring. How do you learn such a profound lesson? Perhaps diabetes itself is the teacher.

Because we believe that diabetes is a teacher about living, we have chosen to make this book more than a manual on testing blood, taking shots, and balancing rutabagas against radishes. Having diabetes is a challenge, a burden, a transformation, a robber, and a blessing. So let's accept its gracious gift and let it teach us to live the years we do have well.

Willing To Live Well

Although a cure for diabetes is probably many years away, fundamental breakthroughs in diabetes care have been made in recent years. These breakthroughs include

- Home blood glucose tests that give immediate and accurate feedback on your blood sugar levels whenever you need it.

- New approaches to the use of insulin that enable you to maintain better control of blood sugar.

- Better information about the steps you can take to reduce the risk of developing diabetic complications.

- Improved treatments for complications, which have allowed thousands of diabetics to save their vision, avoid impotence, survive kidney disease, and reduce the effects of heart disease.

- Greater awareness of the emotional and behavioral implications of diabetes.

- New knowledge about nutrition and diet.

- Recognition of diabetes education as a lifelong learning experience.

These are significant improvements and ones that may enable you to normalize many of your body functions (such as blood sugar, blood fats, cholesterol, and hormones). There is strong evidence that controlling blood sugar levels and other aspects of body chemistry greatly reduces the risk of developing diabetic complications. Studies are underway to test this hypothesis further.

The tightest level of diabetic self-care now available may enable you to keep blood sugar levels close to the normal range. Achieving this highly desirable goal requires that you learn and follow the most demanding regimen medicine offers (what we and others call the *Intensive Regimen*). More modest levels of control still call for education and the willingness to use what you learn.

LEARNING TO DO WHAT YOU CHOOSE TO DO

It is likely that you will have to change some of your behaviors—begin new ones or stop doing old ones. Research has shown that individuals usually progress through five stages when they make major changes in behavior: precontemplation, contemplation, preparation, action, and maintenance. Insight into where you are in the process can help you make realistic plans for change, so we'll briefly outline these stages. (For further information, see the article "In Search of How People Change" by J.O. Prochaska, C.C. DiClemente, and J.C. Norcross in the September 1992 issue of *American Psychologist*. The article focuses mostly on addictive behaviors related to smoking, eating, and alcohol because most research is about them, but the stages apply to any kind of difficult-to-change behaviors.)

- Precontemplation is the stage during which there is no intention to change behavior in the foreseeable future (e.g., six months). Wishing to change is different from seriously intending to change.

- Contemplation is the stage where you are aware of a behavior you want to change and are seriously thinking about doing it but have not yet made a commitment to act. This stage can last a long time (knowing where you want to go but not quite ready to get started).

- The preparation stage combines intention to act with some initial preliminary steps (e.g., preparing a daily log sheet, buying a home blood glucose meter.)

- The action stage is where it happens. It takes a considerable commitment of time, energy, and effort.

- Finally, maintenance is the stage where the individual works to prevent return to old behaviors and incorporate the changes into a regular, habitual mode of action.

Most of us don't move in a straight line through these stages—rather we may spiral back into a preceding stage or stages, each spiral getting us further along until we are finally successful in the maintenance stage.

It's important for you to recognize where you are in these stages, so you can be realistic about your expectations and not berate your-self if progress is slower or less direct than you would like. The items on the list below will help you focus on the change processes needed to move through the stages.

If you have had diabetes for some time, some items on this list are probably a part of your life already. Adding others may make living with diabetes much easier for you. You might check off the ones you already practice and note those you would like to add. Later, if you encounter difficulties, it may help you to see if something from this list offers a solution.

1. Believe that treatment for diabetes is effective. If you doubt that this is so, try to understand the basis for your doubt.

2. Recognize that diabetes is a serious condition worthy of your respect, even if it presents few symptoms at present.

3. Balance seriousness with lightness, humor, and detachment.

4. Believe that you are capable of learning and following any regimen you adopt.

5. Recognize that you are the one who chooses how you will care for yourself. Make your choices consciously.

6. Make decisions about diabetes self-care in the context of your other life needs. Don't neglect other important aspects of your life or the overall quality of your life.

7. In choosing how you will care for yourself, find a balance between your subjective preferences and your objective needs.

8. Watch your stress level as you work on diabetes care. Use stress-management tools to keep the experience from becoming an additional source of strain.

9. Offer yourself healthful rewards for both your efforts and achievements. Recognize what feels better is itself a reward for improved self-care.

10. Define the tasks required by the regimen you choose. Divide the tasks and the behavioral changes into small, concrete steps. Set goals so you understand clearly what will demonstrate your success. Create a realistic time schedule for the learning or change.

11. Explore possible difficulties you may encounter in the process of change you are entering. Plan ways of dealing with them in advance.

12. Make a solid commitment to changing your behavior and learning the new skills and information you need.

13. When you feel reluctant to take on a particular change, try it for a short, predetermined time and see how it affects your life.

14. Give yourself positive feedback as you learn and support yourself when you have difficulty learning. Don't cling to feelings of guilt or failure.

15. When obstacles arise, deal with them and learn from them.

16. Evaluate your efforts and achievements objectively, without self-condemnation.

We will briefly discuss each of these factors affecting learning and sticking with your self-care program. Why are they important? What is there about diabetes that makes them especially relevant?

1. Believe that treatment for diabetes is effective. If you doubt that this is so, try to understand the basis for your doubt.

Obviously, if you don't believe treatment will do much good, you will have difficulty sticking with any regimen. This issue becomes complex with diabetes. As we have said, there is no guarantee that excellent self-care will prevent long-term complications. Effective treatment is a matter of improving your odds, but you cannot eliminate the risk of developing complications.

However, when you improve blood sugar control to moderate or tight levels, you get a short-term demonstration of effectiveness: You feel better, both mentally and physically.

Gary's Experience

> *"As my control improves, I feel leaner and healthier. I'm less sluggish, as though my blood has become less viscous with the reduction of excess sugar. I sleep better because I don't have to get up two or three times a night to go to the bathroom.*
>
> *I was concerned that I might become preoccupied with diabetes as I tightened up my control. Actually, I find I can be less aware of it because there are fewer symptoms of high blood sugar to remind me."*

If you choose loose control, you may still experience the short-term disadvantages of high blood sugar, depending on how high your tests run. But there is a level of effectiveness even here. By maintaining a limited regimen and remaining committed to learning more from it, you keep a positive attitude. You will be in a better position to improve physical control if and when you choose to.

2. Recognize that diabetes is a serious condition worthy of your respect, even if it presents few symptoms at present.

When you exercise a moderate degree of control, you may experience few symptoms of diabetes. Even when blood sugar levels are fairly high, it is possible to grow accustomed to the short-term symptoms: thirst, frequent urination, sluggishness, and susceptibility to infection and illness.

Unless complications develop, it's not easy to feel the seriousness of diabetes through your direct experience with it. Unlike people with arthritis, for instance, you have few immediate and painful reminders. You have to create your own personal way of remembering that diabetes is a crucial aspect of your life.

Respecting Diabetes

Writing your thoughts down can help you define the significance of diabetes in your life. Answer the questions spontaneously, even if the ideas that first come to mind seem inappropriate.

1. What aspects of diabetes make it a serious condition, one that may have a major impact on your life?

2. Do you ever feel you have no future because of diabetes?

3. Do you avoid looking at problems and difficulties that arise because of your diabetes?

4. Do you sometimes take diabetes too seriously? If so, how?

5. Do you have any doubts about the long-term significance of diabetes? If so, quickly scan Chapter 17, where complications are described.

3. Balance seriousness with lightness, humor, and detachment.

Diabetes is, at this point, a lifelong companion. You might as well make it an agreeable one, threats and all.

You can invoke lightness and humor when you are in a difficult spot by telling the story of your serious situation as though you were speaking of a third person, someone you are fond of but whom you find gently amusing. (You might even try telling the story to the person in the mirror.) Or look back from a decade in the future. See yourself and your dilemmas from a time when you have long since resolved them. Note the clever ways you avoided seeing the obvious solutions back then.

The detachment we speak of here is not indifference, but rather a viewing of yourself and the problems you face from a larger perspective. From this point of view, you are not attached to the feelings and beliefs that often appear to trap you. You experience and acknowledge them, but you realize that you are more than these limitations. You can draw on your full resources to break through the limits.

Humor is a powerful way of breaking attachments. When you can laugh at habitual behavior, you feel less allegiance to it.

4. Believe that you are capable of learning and following any regimen you adopt.

Feeling competent may come naturally to you, or you may be one of the many people who learned to doubt that you can do what you set out to do. *Learned* is the key word here. Whether your doubts stem from feeling you are dumb, contrary, or stuck for life, they are aspects of self-image that you can unlearn. Diabetes itself tends to make us feel like dummies, even when we have no difficulties with learning or changing in other areas. This was especially true before the recent breakthroughs in self-care.

Ernest's Experience

"Out of 44 years of living with diabetes, I spent 30 of them resolving to try to make an effort to get it under control. I thought I knew what I should do. Actually doing it seemed harder than climbing Mount Everest. For one thing, I didn't feel I could ask my doctor for help. That would mean I'd have to tell him how out of control I was! At least I always tried to look like a good patient.

So I'd study my 1954 Joslin's Diabetes Manual. I'd measure the food I ate. I'd pee in the test tube. And I'd get more and more uptight. Nothing made any sense to me. I couldn't predict when I would or would not spill sugar. What an incredible sense of frustration and failure came with that stinking orange color foaming up at me in the test tube!

Of course, I always felt that I'd done something wrong, no matter how hard I'd tried. No one had ever mentioned that emotional stress affects blood sugar levels strongly; or that the *urine test is very imprecise, measuring only moderately high, very high, and very very high; or that one shot a day of intermediate insulin couldn't possibly prevent large ups and downs in blood sugar level.*

In short, I didn't know that I was in a double bind, being expected to do something but not having the tools necessary to do it. It was like being asked to build a house with bent nails and a hammer without a handle and feeling incompetent because the task seemed impossible."

Today the diabetes tool kit is full of new tools for both physical and psychological self-care, but diabetes is still not necessarily easy to master. If you choose to work for the tightest level of control, your ability to learn and to change behavior will be challenged. And even with the best effort, in some cases a moderate level of control is the best that can be achieved because of hormonal factors or high levels of stress.

Whenever you achieve less than your goal, don't label yourself a failure. Give yourself credit for what you have achieved, and look to see what you still have to learn or change to reach your goal. (This may be something other than what you set out to learn.) With this point of view, you learn from whatever happens, and you continue to believe in your capacity to learn. (Chapter 14, "Living Well With Yourself," contains ideas on freeing yourself from the limits described here.)

5. Recognize that you are the one who chooses how you will care for yourself. Make your choices consciously.

Your doctor, nurse, dietitian, social worker, or diabetes educator cannot make the actual choices for you. Only you can make them. You are the only one who can integrate prescriptions, recommendations, and external pressures into your life.

Sometimes you may find it difficult to accept the responsibility of making choices, especially when the choices conflict with professional recommendations. Then it is easier to say, "I don't have time to do all this testing," or "The cafeteria doesn't have the right kind of food for my diet," or "It's too much hassle to test my blood when I'm at work," or "I carry enough stuff around with me already."

If you make your choices consciously and accept them, you gain power. ("I prefer to sleep an extra few minutes rather than get up to test," or "I don't want to bother fixing a bag lunch.") You also make clear to yourself what the alternatives are, and you may find it easier to make more healthful decisions.

As we said at the beginning of this book, the realization of your power to choose all aspects of your regimen is fundamental to your following it. Your life is under your control. You make the important decisions. If you rebel against your own authority, then learning to stop doing that simply becomes one more item on your learning agenda.

Your medical team can do more than recommend a self-care program. Your physician and other professionals can also help you understand the alternatives available to you, and you can ask them to work with you on identifying and overcoming barriers you encounter. Don't be afraid to say, "That's going to be hard for me to do because . . . ." In fact, they'll appreciate it.

6. Make decisions about diabetes self-care in the context of your other life needs. Don't neglect other important aspects of your life or the overall quality of your life.

Health professionals naturally place top priority on your diabetes care and may even forget that you have other concerns. Diabetes itself sometimes urgently demands that you deal with it before all else. But most of the time, you must balance your needs as a diabetic with a host of other issues. If you don't, you may run into difficulties in many areas of your life. Use the following table to catalog your various needs and sort out your priorities.

In the following table, note specific important needs in any of the areas on the left, then use the other categories to help you rank them according to the amount of attention they demand from you.

	Specific Need
Diabetes Care	
Work	
Family	
Leisure	
Other Issues	
Education and Intellectual Growth	
Spiritual Concerns	

If this exercise suggests that you have enough concerns to keep a whole regiment busy, don't despair. See what can possibly be postponed or dealt with gradually. Reserve at least a few minutes each day to improving your diabetes care. Then set a date to review your priorities in a month or two.

Often several needs can be satisfied by a single, well-chosen activity. Dancing or sports, for instance, can help you improve metabolic control while providing enjoyment and social interaction. Better relations with your spouse and mutual support around diabetes issues could both be served by participation in a support group or communications workshop. When you find connections between your different needs in this way, you won't spend nearly as much time dealing with them separately.

7. In choosing how you will care for yourself, find a balance between your subjective preferences and objective needs.

16

Actions Called For	Difficulty	Urgency	Rank

You can't ignore your feelings, but you also can't let them dominate your decisions about self-care. The best choices come out of an inner dialogue between your emotional and rational sides, with intuition helping. This dialogue may happen spontaneously with you, or you may need a structure to guide your decision making.

One simple way of opening this inner dialogue is to write it out, with your emotional self discussing the issue in question with your rational self.

8. Watch your stress level as you work on diabetes care. Use stress-management tools to keep the experience from becoming an additional source of strain.

It is possible to work at learning diabetes care with so much anxiety and tension that blood sugar levels shoot up solely because of the stress you are generating. In this area of your life, it is especially important for you to work with an awareness of the cues of stress. Let your body remind you when it's time to slow down and relax. (Chapter 11 contains many techniques for dealing with stress.)

9. Offer yourself healthful rewards for both your efforts and achievements. Recognize that feeling better is itself a reward for improved self-care.

Rewards are a very important part of diabetes care because our condition deprives us of some old pleasures. People often reward themselves with sweets or extra food, for instance, but for people with diabetes, this is a penalty, not a prize. You may benefit from creating a positive reward system to offset possible feelings of deprivation.

As you work on learning and changing behavior, rewards also help reinforce the effort you make and the changes you achieve. The most substantial rewards, of course, come from feeling better physically, and from feeling more powerful and optimistic mentally. But there is good evidence that additional bonuses help keep motivation high.

Take a few minutes now to jot down a variety of rewards you would appreciate: gifts, good times, experiences, or even things it would be nice *not* to do. Then, at the start of any particular diabetes learning project, promise yourself one reward for effort after a certain period and another reward when you have successfully completed the learning project.

You May Have Already Won...

1. Gifts I can give myself: _____

_____

2. Celebrations and other good times I'd enjoy: _____

_____

3. New experiences I would value: _____

_____

4. Some things I'd like not to have to do: _____

_____

---

10. Define the tasks required by the regimen you choose. Divide the tasks and the behavior changes into small, concrete steps. Set goals so you understand clearly what will demonstrate your success. Create a realistic time schedule for the learning or change.

It may seem to you that learning to manage diabetes is a full-time job. That's why this item is so important. When you divide a large project into its individual steps and schedule the steps over a realistic period, the project seems—and becomes—much more manageable. Make the first step in particular a small and easy one. However much urgency you may feel, you simply cannot learn it all yesterday. Once you have mastered the basic survival skills (detecting and treating reactions, taking your shot, dealing with infections and illness, etc.), you can proceed with other learning and changing at a reasonable pace.

By setting reasonable and specific goals, you give yourself a much better chance of experiencing success as you progress. If you have been very poorly controlled, saying "I'll get my diabetes under control sometime" is too vague. Aiming at an average blood test of 180 milligrams of glucose per deciliter of blood (mg/dl) in a month gives you a manageable target, and you will clearly know whether you have attained it.

11. Explore possible difficulties you may encounter in the process of change you are entering. Plan ways of dealing with them in advance.

You may be one of the blessed who never have trouble doing anything. Or you may be like most of us, sometimes running into blocks. If the latter is true, you probably know what your typical difficulties are and ways you have dealt with them in the past. By making some notes on escape routes at the beginning, you will be able to draw on more creativity than you usually have available when you hit a stumbling block.

TROUBLE SPOTS

In the past, I have gotten stuck learning or following a diabetes regimen because_____

_____

I have run into trouble in areas other than diabetes because

_____

I have moved (or could move) through the difficulty by_____

_____

---

12. Make a solid commitment to changing your behavior and learning the new skills and information you need.

For some people, the matter of commitment falls into place easily, without being formalized. But others like to state their intentions in a way that helps them strengthen their will to change, in some cases even making a contract with themselves. If this appeals to you, you can use the following form.

A Contract with Myself

I commit myself to changing this behavior or learning this aspect of diabetes care (be as specific as possible):_____

_____

I believe this will improve my diabetes self-care by_____

_____

I believe I am capable of doing this, although I may need assistance in the form of _____

_____

If I experience difficulties in completing this task, I will use the help processes in Chapter 3 to help me overcome them.

I will learn from the whole experience—setbacks as well as achievements.

(Optional)

I will receive the following reward for effort by (specific date)

_____

I will receive the following reward for achievement upon completion _____

_____

If I do not fulfill this contract I will (specify penalty)_____

_____

I can reasonably expect to complete this by _____

Signature_____

Date_____

13. When you feel reluctant to take on a particular change, try it for a short, predetermined time and see how it affects your life.

Some alterations in life-style suggested by diabetes may arouse resistance in you. When this happens, it helps to remember that we often tend to exaggerate the consequences of changes we don't wish to make. In our imagination, we see only the negative and blow that up to monumental proportions.

If you tend to do this, you can suspend negative expectations and do a trial run. For instance, test your blood sugar four times a day for a few days, if that's what you're resisting. (Even a commitment of a day at a time can help.) In this case, make no commitment beyond that period. Then contrast what you actually experience with your prior expectations. Whatever the specific change is, you are likely to find it's not as bad as you thought it would be.

(If you still have trouble beginning, see if you can break the task down into smaller steps and try just the first step for a while, then try the second, and so forth.)

14. Give yourself positive feedback as you learn, and support yourself when you have difficulty learning. Don't cling to feelings of guilt or failure.

Just having diabetes is enough of an emotional load. You don't have to make it a bigger burden by telling yourself you are a "bad" diabetic. You improve your willingness to manage the illness well by accepting yourself when you have trouble learning about or following a regimen.

As you learn, notice the improvements, the changes, and the efforts you make, and consciously acknowledge them. Don't ignore your mistakes or your tendencies to hold back, but observe them without blame. They are simply areas requiring further attention. (Chapter 14, "Living Well With Yourself," includes ideas for supporting yourself and dealing with guilt.)

15. When obstacles arise, deal with them and learn from them.

An obstacle that you can't seem to push through is really a new learning assignment. Say you have started to learn home blood testing, but you are afraid to prick your finger, even with one of the automatic devices. Then your new assignment is learning to deal with fear of physical discomfort or negative expectations or whatever is at work in you.

Or perhaps the obstacle is total resistance to learning about diabetic complications. You break into a cold sweat every time you think of looking at that subject. In this case, you recognize an opportunity to learn about your feelings of vulnerability or mortality. Before—and probably while—studying complications, you need to work with these very human emotions. Perhaps you could enlist a friend or relative to help. Other diabetics who have dealt with these issues can also give valuable support.

16. Evaluate your efforts and achievements objectively, without self-condemnation.

Each time you complete an aspect of your diabetes learning program, take a moment to evaluate your work in a nonjudgmental manner. Look at both how you worked on it and what you accomplished. Give yourself credit for what you did achieve, even when you have not yet reached your final goal. Be honest with yourself about the shortcomings of your work, but don't view the shortcomings as a sign of weakness.

This clear process of evaluation is especially important in learning to manage diabetes well. Our condition demands a great deal from us. There are many variables affecting diabetic control. Sometimes we can make the best possible effort and still find blood sugar outside the limits we try to attain. It is important not to add negative judgments to the frustrations we naturally feel. If we are to continue with the project, we must congratulate ourselves for hanging in there and look carefully to see what to do next.

Living Well At The Beginning of Diabetes

> **"I** really felt sorry for myself [when I found out I had diabetes]. I still want to know 'Why me?' I never did anything to deserve this. Why all of a sudden do I have to stick to a diet and take shots for the rest of my life?"
>
> — *Carol, 17 years old*
> (*In* Focus on Feelings, *Pyramid Films*)

If you have only recently discovered that you have diabetes, take a deep breath, sigh, and relax for a moment. You are going through a crisis. You may be handling the challenges of this time well, or you may feel overwhelmed by them. In either case, it is a difficult, demanding situation, and you need all the breaks you can get.

At the beginning of diabetes, you have three basic demands to handle:

1. *Practical tasks.* You must learn new skills, absorb new information, make decisions, and change aspects of the way you live.

2. *Emotional tasks.* You need to deal with the emotional impact of being told that you have a lifelong chronic disease that as yet has no cure.

3. *Support tasks*. You need to mobilize internal and external sources of support.

You may find yourself trying to meet all three needs at the same time, as well as dealing with the other needs in your life. It is very easy to feel overloaded in this initial period. So remember, *you can't do everything at once*. Set priorities, with the help of your doctor and the medical staff.

PRACTICAL TASKS

The practical demands of diabetes begin very quickly, much sooner than you feel ready for them. Even if you have gone into the hospital to get your system under control, you soon find that you are not allowed to play the role of the passive patient. You realize your life depends on learning a dizzying amount of information very quickly. Your learning may be marked by a bit of anxiety, since it is difficult to understand initially which information is of life-or-death importance. You are still dealing with the emotional shock of the diagnosis, as well as with the physical stress of diabetes out of control, so your mind may be functioning with less clarity than usual.

This is an excellent time to learn the fundamental lesson of diabetes education: When you don't understand something or when you feel overloaded with information, tell your doctor firmly and clearly. Ask for a restatement or a pause. Don't just nod your head so the doctor won't think you are stupid. Some health professionals are very good communicators, but others don't notice if you are suffering from information overload.

Sometimes your physician will involve other health professionals. In this case, your basic care will be supervised by the doctor, but the specific educational aspects may be handled by a nurse, dietitian or diabetes educator.

Acute Versus Chronic Health Care

Until recently, newly diagnosed diabetics were usually hospitalized to get their blood sugar under control. Now this process is often accomplished through office visits and phone contact, so long as the initial symptoms are not too extreme. In either case, you will experience a combination of acute and chronic medical care, which may be confusing.

Before beginning treatment for diabetes, many people know only acute care. Acute care is that in which a doctor steps in to deal with a short-term illness or some other emergency. A patient in this situation usually has relatively little involvement other than following a few instructions. At the beginning of diabetes, your physician has to act quickly to restore order to a system seriously out of control.

But from the very beginning in diabetes, your doctor and the other health professionals are initiating you to a radically different style of medicine: chronic medical self-care. You are given extensive training to take care of yourself for the rest of your life. Within a few years, health professionals may be telling you that you know more than they do about diabetes. They are there to assist you in this process and to take charge when an acute crisis (such as diabetic coma) occurs. But you are the only one who can be responsible for your day-to-day care.

Your Treatment Program

Being in charge of your diabetes care may seem to be an enormous responsibility at first, but hundreds of thousands of diabetics assume it and live well every year. Your medical team will provide lots of hand holding in the beginning, so you can always call for help when you can't figure out what to do. If you have some other diabetics to consult on the many smaller practical questions that arise, you can avoid feeling that you are bothering your medical team with too many queries.

If you feel able to meet the challenge, there are strong arguments for adopting an intensive treatment program right at the beginning. This will be the most intense period of diabetes learning you will go through. What you learn in the beginning tends to stick with you for years. If you begin with a fairly loose level of management, you may have a hard time tightening up on your regimen later. Maintaining excellent patterns of self-care from the first also strengthens your chances of benefiting from any future advances in research, such as islet cell transplants.

Some people are able to begin diabetes self-care at this level very easily. Others feel too overwhelmed by the shock of diagnosis to begin with such a detailed program. If you feel it is more than you can handle at this time, start with a more moderate regimen, but think of it as a temporary decision. When you have adjusted to the initial demands of diabetes, reconsider the intensive regimen.

Another factor affecting the standard of care you adopt at the beginning is the experience and attitude of your physician. As a whole, the profession is moving toward tighter control, but there is still a great variety of opinions on this matter. If you wish to maintain fairly strict control and your doctor doesn't strongly support this choice, you may need to find one who does. On the other hand, if your physician urges strict control and you do not feel ready for it, you can probably negotiate for looser control. Create a plan for moving in the direction your doctor recommends over the next few months. If a difference of opinion remains, you may need to find a new doctor.

Diabetes: A Lifelong Learning Experience

Living well with diabetes requires learning well for the rest of your life. You have probably already started discovering what a powerful teacher diabetes is, with its many challenges and surprises. You are in the midst of absorbing many practical details of care, some of which have life-or-death significance. At this stage, you need to determine which aspects of care have such vital importance. (See "Diabetes Survival Kit" at the back of the book.) You are probably changing aspects of your lifestyle and you are dealing with (or avoiding) the emotions that occur when diabetes is diagnosed.

Diabetes treatment is continually evolving, so you can expect to continue learning about it for many years. As you grow older, you may find that you are learning some of life's important lessons sooner and more deeply than your nondiabetic friends. Our physical condition calls on us to make peace with vulnerability and mortality and to value the preciousness of life. The depth of experience that accompanies such learning can be seen as a powerful benefit of this condition.

Learning About Diabetes

To avoid feeling overwhelmed by the amount you have to learn in the first months of diabetes, divide the learning into manageable lessons. Work out a time schedule. Identify the resources that can assist you. There may be a series of classes at a local hospital or clinic. A diabetes educator (usually a nurse or dietitian) may be available. Your local chapter of the American Diabetes Association may offer educational programs and support groups. Don't worry if you find that your doctor seems to play a relatively minor role in the educational process. In many cases, other members of your health care team will have more time and training in this field.

EMOTIONAL TASKS

Ask a dozen of us how we reacted to being told we have diabetes and you will probably hear a dozen different stories: "It really scared me. My uncle had diabetes and he died when he was 40." "No big deal. I don't let things like that get to me." "I was angry for months. I thought it would destroy all of my plans." "I just pulled the covers over my head and felt numb."

There is no "right" way to feel, only the way you are feeling. Give yourself time, in the midst of learning countless practical details, to experience your particular emotions. If your style is to deal with feelings on your own, be sure you set aside periods to do this. Some people use writing, some take long solitary walks, others pray or meditate. (See Chapter 14, "Living Well With Yourself," for ways of handling your feelings.)

If you prefer to have assistance, remember that it is available, even if you think you are relatively isolated. There may be people available in your present support network; if not, you have guaranteed membership in the community of people with diabetes. Some people may also find value in a few sessions with a counselor, psychologist, or social worker.

Some common reactions to being told you are diabetic are described in the following paragraphs. To some extent, these feelings can be countered by information at a rational level, but you may find that the feeling persists even when you "know better." It may be simply your familiar way of reacting to situations—an old habit. The section on emotions in Chapter 14 offers means of dealing with some emotional habits.

You may feel helpless or unable to assume the new responsibilities diabetes assigns to you. With this response, it helps to discuss your feelings with other diabetics. Their reassurance comes from knowing that these feelings of being overwhelmed diminish as you actually start taking care of yourself.

You may be *depressed, fearful,* or *angry* over the many changes in lifestyle you are expected to achieve. Some of the changes are specific to diabetes, but it is useful to recognize that the majority of them are the basics of healthful living for anyone. Regular exercise and a balanced, moderate diet are the requirements of any human body. Even the scheduling required by diabetes can be much more flexible now, with multiple daily insulin injections or the insulin pump.

Perhaps you are *anxious* or *depressed* over the possibility of developing complications and dying early. Grim stories and statistics of the casualties of diabetes may lead you to believe you are doomed to disability and an early grave. Actually, recent advances in diabetes care offer the means of preventing or delaying the onset of diabetic complications. (See Chapters 15-17, "Living Well With Complications.")

You may feel *frustrated* over the changes in life goals you believe diabetes imposes. Actually, diabetes closes very few doors to you. You are not allowed to fly a plane solo. You would probably find it impossible to get some jobs where an insulin reaction would threaten the safety of others. But most roles you might seek are open to you, including the role of mother or father.

One reaction to diabetes that may appear completely positive is doing everything right, but *doing it with so much anxiety* that you feel terrible. If you are caught in this pattern, make relaxation and other stress management techniques a high priority. You will also benefit from sorting out which aspects of diabetes care are most critical. Until you do this, the slightest mistake in self-care may seem threatening.

The opposite reaction is to be *unconcerned,* insisting that diabetes will have no effect whatsoever on your life. At some level, you may even believe that you don't really have the disease. Once you get your blood sugar under a moderate degree of control, diabetes has few outward signs. What a "nice" disease it seems to be. The temptation to do as little as possible to control it may be strong, especially when you seem to be getting away with "murder." In type I diabetes, there is even a "honeymoon period," a few months during which insulin requirements temporarily decrease. However, after this period, they do go up again.

Living well with diabetes calls for accepting it as a fact of life, a fact of major significance. The more you try to ignore it through minimal self-care, the greater the impact it can have. If, on the other hand, you follow a full regimen, you will lessen the risks and ensure that your body will be in shape to benefit from future advances in treatment or a cure.

SUPPORT TASKS

At the beginning of diabetes, you can find strong support for dealing with both the practical and the emotional issues. Relatives, friends, other diabetics, and professionals may be called upon at this time. You may need comfort, encouragement, or honest feedback on how you are handling things. You may have hundreds of questions that seem too minor to take to your doctor. You may need information on cutting the costs of the supplies you need.

Some people know that they are blessed with abundant support networks at times like this. Others feel isolated and don't know where to turn. If you tend to feel there is little support available to you, give yourself a chance to be surprised. You may have more resources than you think. Even if you know few people, you are probably no more than two or three phone calls away from dozens of people who are ready and willing to help you cope.

Wherever you live, there are other people nearby with diabetes who are well informed, positive, and helpful. You can make contact with other diabetics through your physician, your pharmacist or other health professionals, through the American Diabetes Association or the Juvenile Diabetes Foundation, or through people you already know. Let them know you are looking for people who have a positive outlook and who don't mind talking with others who have diabetes. If you encounter people who only like to complain or tell horror stories, steer clear of them. You need support, not discouragement. (See Chapter 13 for more on networking.)

Beginning Well

This questionnaire is designed to help you bring order to the process of adjusting to diabetes. Use your answers here to guide you in sorting out your new priorities. See what requests you need to make of your health care team and support network. What immediate changes do you need to make in your own life to help you handle this crisis well? If the challenge of diabetes feels overwhelming, identify small first steps you know you can handle. The most important thing is getting started.

1. *Your Support Network*

    The people I can count on for emotional support include _____

    _____

    The people who will help me with practical problems (getting to an appointment with the doctor, bringing food when I'm ill, etc.) include _____

    _____

    (If you have trouble asking for help) I wouldn't want to ask for help because _____

    _____

    How would you answer a friend who gave you this reason?____

    _____

(If you feel you need more support) I can enlarge my support network by:

_____ Contacting the American Diabetes Association or the Juvenile Diabetes Foundation.

_____ Joining a support group (either general or diabetic).

_____ Asking my minister for help.

_____ Asking my doctor or pharmacist to help me get in touch with other people with diabetes.

_____ Going to a social worker or psychologist.

_____ Other. _____

(If there are people in your life who are discouraging or otherwise negative) I can neutralize this "antisupport" by

_____ Asking the person involved to change.

_____ Changing how I respond.

_____ Avoiding the person.

_____ Having more contact with people who show a positive attitude.

_____ Other. _____

The personal strengths I can call on within myself at this time include _____

_____

A past crisis I handled well was _____

_____

2. *Your Physical Care*

_____ I know which aspects of diabetes management have life-or-death significance. (See "Diabetes Survival Kit" at back of book.)

_____ I feel satisfied with my physician.

_____ I feel my physician is adequate, but I would like him/her to

_____

_____

_____ I feel I need a different doctor because _____

_____

I feel most certain about the aspects of diabetes care I've checked below:

_____ Insulin dosage

_____ Insulin reactions

_____ Blood testing

_____ Urine testing

_____ Diet and meal planning

_____ Exercise

_____ The effect of stress on control of diabetes

_____ The interactions among all of these

(If your budget is limited) Have you located the least expensive source for diabetes supplies? A local ADA chapter might be able to refer you to medical discount shopping services. Or refer to the Appendix.

3. *Your Emotional Care*

My emotional reactions to the diagnosis of diabetes include the items I've checked below:

_____ Anger

_____ Fear

_____ Anxiety

_____ Depression

_____ Guilt

_____ Lack of feeling

_____ Calm

_____ Other

I am dealing with these reactions by _____

_____

My overall response to the diagnosis of diabetes includes the items I've checked below:

_____ I feel overwhelmed by the whole thing and find it difficult to handle.

_____ I am upset because I have to make too many changes in my life.

_____ I feel anxious about the things I have heard about complications.

_____ I am concerned the diabetes will make it impossible to achieve my life goals.

_____ I am very worried about doing all the diabetes procedures right.

_____ I have withdrawn into myself.

_____ I don't believe that diabetes is any big deal or that I have to change much.

_____ I am dealing well with my feelings and with the practical challenges that diabetes has presented.

_____ Other _____

I can reduce the negative side of my overall response to diabetes by _____

_____

_____

4. *Your Diabetes Learning Program*

____ I have a good sense of what I know and what I still have to learn.

____ I feel confused and need help figuring out what is important to learn.

____ I have enrolled in a diabetes instruction class.

____ I have subscribed to

____ *Diabetes Forecast*

____ *Diabetes Self-Management*

____ *Diabetes in the News*

(See Appendix for addresses.)

Review your answers and put 1, 2 or 3 stars by them to indicate their importance to you. Use this ranking to guide your use of this book.

C H A P T E R 3

Help!

You may have noticed there are times when life gets difficult. And then diabetes has a way of adding its distinctive difficulties to those we already face as human beings. Our self-care regimen is demanding both to learn and to practice. We meet a variety of unique health crises, both immediate and long term. We are threatened by insulin reactions, delayed meals, lost insulin, forgotten injections, coma, runaway infections, depression, anxiety, denial, difficulties in relationships, and an amazing array of diabetic complications. Yes, there are times when life gets difficult.

You may have come to this chapter because you are in one of those times. You may be in the midst of a diabetes crisis and need help handling your feelings and actions. Or you may feel unable (or unwilling) to continue learning what you need to know to care for yourself well. Here you will find a number of tools to help you understand what is happening. You will also find what you need to do to move on.

While you can do much to help yourself, you may need help from your medical team or personal support network. Don't be afraid to give yourself permission to ask for that help. *If the specific crisis you are handling is an aspect of your physical care, do not fail to call your doctor or nurse practitioner for help.*

We offer a variety of methods to suit different individual styles and situations. You may want to work through the whole sequence laid out here, or you may need to use only one or two of the methods. Choose the course that is right for you.

We recommend beginning with relaxation and detachment. This will help you gain perspective and work more effectively.

TOOLS FOR RESCUING YOURSELF FROM A CRISIS

Relaxation

When you have trouble—especially when your health is at stake—a natural response is to become uptight and frustrated. The more tense you become, the harder it is to see a way out. You get tunnel vision when you're nervous, anxious, or scared. So you are wise to begin the process of rescuing yourself by relaxing as deeply as possible before doing anything more. This will broaden your vision.

If you have healthful techniques for relaxing that work for you, use them. Eating, drinking, watching television, and other common distractions don't count as healthful techniques. You may already be using practices described at the end of the chapter on stress management or ones that you learned elsewhere.

If you need a new means of relaxing right now, try this:

- Begin by slowly saying something like: "My only job right now is to relax." For the moment, put all other concerns aside.

- Then, focus awareness on your breath, especially the feeling of it as you exhale. You can even sigh as you breathe out, if you like.

- Your body will respond now, if you talk with it. Say, "My right arm is growing heavier." Repeat it slowly in your mind, four or five times, or as many times as it takes to feel heavier.

- Now, repeat the same thing for your left arm: "My left arm is growing heavier," then your right leg, and after that, your left leg.

- Within five to ten minutes, the feeling of heaviness you are describing will have been translated by your body into a greater sense of relaxation. You can help the process by focusing your mind on whatever heaviness develops as you go along, rather than on the tensions that remain.

If you are familiar with spiritual practices, prayer or meditation may be the most effective means of relaxation you can use. These practices may also help you gain insight into the problem you are dealing with. Learn to pay attention to that kind, supportive voice inside you guiding you toward better health decisions. (Other techniques of relaxation are described at the end of Chapter 11, "Living Well With Stress.")

Detachment

When difficulties arise, we often feel closed in, limited. We lose both clear perception and creativity because we are so focused on what is wrong. Finding solutions is much easier if we can gain some distance from the difficult situation. This is especially true when a great deal is at stake, as with a pregnant woman trying to gain optimal control over diabetes, or with someone who has major diabetes complications developing. No matter how urgent the need to achieve a particular goal, it is more likely to be attained if the sense of anxious need can be suspended.

Following are a few of the many ways you might gain detachment from your reactions in a difficult situation. Once you have the basic idea, you will probably be able to find a way particularly suited to your style.

- Adopt an attitude of curiosity. Look at your situation as an artist or scientist who says, "Hmmm, very interesting. Let me explore what is happening."

- Remember a time of success, a time when things were going well for you, or when you felt very calm and peaceful. See or feel the places, happenings, or people that were part of this special time. Let the remembrance of positive feelings come into the present, reminding you that you are more than someone having a problem.

- Think of another area of your present life in which you are successful. Appreciate the strengths and skills that you demonstrate here. Imagine what it would mean to act with these qualities on the problem you are now facing.

- Speak in the past tense when describing the difficulties you are working on now. Look back on them from a time in the future when they have all been overcome and you have made great progress. See this immediate time as only one of many steps you needed to take to reach your goal.

- Describe your problems as those of someone else, someone you care for and understand and whom you see very clearly. Give this person credit for the effort he or she has made and assurance that the challenge will be met.

- Find a humorous point of view for perceiving the situation you are in. Laughter is itself a healing agent as well as a good lubricant for the imagination.

Central to this idea of detachment is letting go of any judgments about yourself and your ability to handle the problem that has arisen. Even if you are dealing with total rebellion against the whole diabetes regimen, suspend the self-condemnation that often goes along with it. You are acting with great power. You just haven't learned how to use that power to support living well.

FINDING OUT WHAT IS GOING ON NOW

You may already have full understanding of what is causing your present crisis and your difficulty in dealing with it. Or you may only have a vague sense of what is happening and why. If you need to develop more awareness of your problem and its source, the following exercise may help you.

Write a brief statement summarizing what you now know about the problem you are facing. This summary will help you clarify the problem and identify the solution. Draw on your answers to any of the following questions in the analysis.

- What are the objective facts of your situation? Which aspects appear to be outside your control? Which ones are within your control?

- When you examine how you are feeling about the problem, what are your strongest emotions? Where in your body do you feel them?

- Consider your thoughts. Are there beliefs or attitudes that make you feel unwilling or unable to deal with this situation? (Typical limiting beliefs here would be: "I can't cope with crisis," "It's too late for me to change," "It's not fair," "I shouldn't have to," "I don't want to."

- In your behavior, what is it that you find difficult to do (or to stop doing)? Break down the behavior into small parts or steps. Figure out which are the most difficult.

- What pictures come to mind when you consider the problem? Do they help you understand what is happening?

- Is there something you are holding onto by having this problem— some positive benefit, such as increased attention from someone you care about?

- Is there something you are avoiding? What undesirable result might come if you were free of this crisis?

- Is something else happening in your life that needs your attention or that is distracting you from what you are trying to accomplish with diabetes?

Some people are most comfortable doing this sort of work on their own, perhaps by writing notes in a journal. Others appreciate talking through a crisis with a friend or relative who is a good listener. A diabetes support group is another good setting for exploring such issues. If no progress is made in any of these ways, a few sessions with a counselor may be in order to sort things out.

CREATING YOUR SOLUTIONS

At times, a clear understanding of what is happening is all that we need to get past an obstacle. "Oh, I was hung up on that old belief 'I'll die by the time I'm 50,' just like Mom. No wonder I was stuck. It's time to get on with learning to live!" When this happens, tension is released and we are restored to full energy.

This may be a time when you need action, not just understanding. If so, take the role of creator, designing the solutions to your present problem. See the situation in its wholeness without blame or judgment. In the work you have just done, identify the specific beliefs, feelings, and behaviors interacting to produce your distress. Then generate a variety of options for dealing with these specifics.

Some guidelines for this process include the following:

- Affirm your ability to handle the situation. Recognize that you choose your responses to what is happening and can make new choices.

- Keep alive to your feelings throughout the process, but do not be trapped by them. Use the techniques for detachment described above when dark feelings seem to dominate. Remember, your feelings are created within you, and you have the power to change them. Ask yourself, "Is this how I want to feel?" If it isn't, create new feelings or attitudes.

- Work with the information about your situation you generated in the previous sections to help define your next steps.

- Identify the specific goals you wish to reach. What changes would let you know you were out of the crisis?

- Brainstorm a list of specific actions that will help you start moving forward. Write down any ideas that come to mind, then search the list for those you feel prepared to take right now. Choose the one that will enable you to take a first step.

- Use your imagination to see or feel yourself taking the actions you need to overcome your problem. In a relaxed state, let scenes unfold in your mind in which you discover new answers. (Also use this visualization to reinforce actions you chose in the previous step.)

- Take a first step, no matter how small. Action restores your confidence to take further action. Action is also an antidote to anxiety.

- Give yourself space for breaks, relaxation, exercise, and entertainment. In most crises, some time off increases your capacity for finding solutions.

If you do everything possible and still feel that you are getting nowhere, look for further help from your health care team and personal support network. Let go of any feeling that you must do this all on your own. Some challenges in living well with diabetes can be met only with outside support.

(See Chapter 14, "Living Well With Yourself," for more on working with feelings and beliefs. Chapter 11, "Living Well With Stress," can also be of aid in a crisis. If you are dealing with the threat or diagnosis of complications, see Section V.)

Section II
LIVING WELL WITH DIABETIC CONTROL

Diabetes—Defining The Choices

Before we developed diabetes, our bodies performed a number of vital functions spontaneously, without our ever having to give a thought to them. The pancreas released insulin whenever it sensed that our blood sugar level was above a certain point. The hormones from other glands kept insulin from lowering blood sugar too much. (These counter-regulatory hormones inhibit insulin action or stimulate the release of sugar into the bloodstream.) We maintained a delicate balance, with blood glucose usually ranging between 60 and 120 mg/dl. We enjoyed a natural control of our sugar metabolism and, as a result, other factors such as blood fats (including cholesterol and triglycerides) remained at normal levels.

When we developed type I diabetes, insulin production from our pancreas was reduced or eliminated. Blood sugar soared to readings two to five times the normal level, or maybe higher. Blood fats increased. Counter-regulatory hormones such as adrenalin—released in flight, fright, fight, or illness—increased because of physical stress and drove our blood sugar levels even higher. Our whole system was out of control.

When we started taking insulin, we regained a semblance of control, but with an enormous difference: *We had to be consciously involved in the metabolic control process.* We had to make decisions about many things that we had never had to worry about before: the amounts of insulin and food to take, the timing of meals and insulin injections, and the effects of exercise or stress on our blood sugar level.

Making metabolic decisions that result in normal blood glucose levels requires information and skill. We need to be able to measure our specific blood sugar level at any moment; we need to know what factors are determining that level (diet, activity, medication, stress, etc.); and we need to know how to vary those factors to regain balance when tests are too high or too low. Finally, we need support—from within or from outside—to maintain the regulated life-style that makes real control of diabetes possible.

Until the last few years, most of us were unable to achieve a good level of control. Only in mild cases of diabetes was it possible to avoid swings in blood sugar level far outside the normal range. Urine tests gave imprecise information about the actual blood glucose level at the time of testing. Once-a-day injections of intermediate or long-acting insulin could not provide the insulin activity needed to handle blood sugar increases after each meal. We knew little about the way emotional stress raises and lowers blood sugar. And the need for emotional support was barely recognized.

All of this has now changed. Home blood glucose testing gives fairly precise readings of blood sugar level any time we need them. An insulin pump or two or more insulin injections each day can provide a supply that more closely matches our hour-to-hour need for insulin. Physicians are encouraging us to learn to make the alterations in insulin dose, diet, and exercise necessary to keep blood glucose levels close to normal. Recognition of the effect of emotional stress on diabetic control has brought a new emphasis on learning means of dealing with stress more effectively; and we are finally admitting the need for emotional support, something required by anyone living with a chronic medical condition.

It is now possible for diabetics who need to develop optimal control rapidly (because of pregnancy, for instance) to do so. Within four or eight weeks, many of us have learned to achieve an average blood sugar level that was impossible five years ago. Even without an urgent short-term need, many of us have gained this level of control simply because we want to live well with diabetes.

The level of regimen needed to maintain optimal control of diabetes is demanding and liberating at the same time. This book outlines a step-by-step process for learning this regimen in an organized and safe fashion. This path is appropriate for people who are prepared to move to a style of intensive diabetes management. This level of management takes commitment, effort, time, a modest amount of money, and close teamwork with your health professionals.

Not everyone is prepared to follow this path. Some people like to move more gradually or are less motivated than others. Some have major concerns other than diabetes competing for their energies. Others may be held back by certain beliefs and emotional reactions that make them feel unable to change. For one reason or another, many diabetics choose to remain at a level of moderate or even loose management.

There are also medical reasons that argue against following this path. The pros and the cons should be weighed in concert with your physician. Because of the increased likelihood of hypoglycemia, patients with significant cardiovascular or cerebrovascular disease might be adding undue risk to an already compromised circulation of nutrients (oxygen and glucose). Patients with "hypoglycemic unawareness"—decreased symptoms due to a variety of reasons that are not now fully understood—are likely to be advised not to follow the intensive regimen. Patients with advanced kidney disease have less predictable insulin action and may find the intensive regimen very difficult to manage.

Although many powerful reasons favor the path of intensive management, we feel it is important not to bias this choice. If diabetics who do not adopt this type of program come to feel that anything less rigorous than the most intensive management is ineffective and futile, they may abandon all efforts to control their metabolism.

You may believe that you have no control at all; your blood sugar levels may soar and plummet crazily. Even so, it is vitally important that you do not condemn yourself as weak or incompetent. By accepting yourself and your past choices, you gain the power to make new, more healthful decisions about self-regulation. If your present choice is a moderate or loose regimen, give yourself credit for what you are doing and continue doing it. You will feel better, and this alone may help you decide to tighten your level of management.

If the Word "Control" Sounds Like Fingernails on a Blackboard...

Most of us believe that living well is living with freedom. Yet when we have diabetes, we are told that we must control our metabolism, our blood sugar, and our eating. Sometimes it seems as though every aspect of our lives requires some kind of control.

There is a basic problem with the word *control* itself. In *Roget's Thesaurus*, the synonyms for control include *whip hand, subjugation, domination, suppression, oppression* and *tyranny.* Verbs associated with control include *browbeat, bully, restrict,* and *corner.* It doesn't sound like a very pleasant place to visit, much less live. No wonder controlling our diabetes often feels like a burden. Yet *control* is one of the most frequently used words in articles on diabetic management, and we have not been able to come up with many adequate substitutes.

We can purge *control* of its negative associations by evoking the image of metabolic order it really represents. When we work to gain control of diabetes, we are seeking deliberately to take over a task our bodies previously handled automatically. If anything, this opportunity of exercising control is a challenge. We are cooperating with and helping direct our life processes. We are not simply managing diabetes; we are managing our lives.

DISCOVERING YOUR PRESENT LEVELS OF CONTROL

We are considering two aspects of control here: the actual level of control you achieve and the level of regimen you follow to control your metabolism. The actual level of control you achieve is measured by home and lab tests and the way you feel. The level of regimen is defined by what you do. Before telling you about the different possible levels,

50

we are going to suggest that you find out about them by determining what your own level is at present. The following questionnaire helps you to do this.

Finding Your Level

Circle the number following the statement that is most true for you. Your doctor's office can supply results of your lab tests if you have had tests done.

A. *Level of Control*

1. My last fasting blood glucose test in the lab or doctor's office was

less than 120 mg/dl	**3**	Don't know or NA	
between 120 and 180	**6**	(not applicable)	
between 181 and 240	**9**		**7.5**
higher than 240	**12**		

2. My last hemoglobin A_1c test was

less than 8%	**3** ✓	higher than 12%	**12**
between 8 and 9.9%	**6**	Don't know or NA	**7.5**
between 10 and 12%	**9**		

3. My last test for total cholesterol was

less than 201	**2**	higher than 240	**8**
between 201 and 225	**4** ✓	Don't know or NA	**5**
between 226 and 240	**6**		

4. The average of all my home blood glucose tests for the last seven days is

less than 120 mg/dl	**2**	higher than 240	**12**
between 120 and 180	**6**	Don't know or NA	**7.5**
between 181 and 240	**9**		

5. The approximate percentage of all my home blood glucose tests
    for the last seven days that were between 60 and 140 mg/dl was

more than 75%	**3**	less than 25%	**12**
between 50 and 75%	**6**	Don't know or NA	**7.5**
between 25 and 50%	**9**		

6. If you do not test blood or urine, or if you do so less than
    twice a week, circle 12 here and skip to question 8.   **12**

7. I test urine for sugar regularly, and I almost never have
    a positive urine test (one or more +).   **2**
    My tests are negative (-) at least half the time and
    usually not higher than 1/4%.   **4**
    My tests vary greatly, sometimes negative, sometimes
    1 or 2%.   **6**
    My tests are usually over 1%.   **8**
    Not applicable, because I test only blood sugar.   **5**

8. When you test for ketones in your urine, the test is

always negative	**2**	frequently positive (1+ times a week)	**8**
always negative unless I am ill or under stress	**4**	NA	**5**
occasionally positive (1-3 times a month)	**6**		

9. I have had severe insulin reactions in the last month
    (severe = strong symptoms such as confusion, shakiness,
    sweating, pounding heart, etc.).

Never	**2**	5-10 times	**6**
1-4 times	**4**	More than 10 times	**8**

10. I have been unconscious from a reaction or failed to
    awaken to a reaction occurring during sleep in the
    last year. If yes, circle 16. If no, skip to question 11.   **16**

11. I have had symptoms of high blood sugar (frequent urination, nighttime urination, thirst, and lethargy) in the last month.

Never	**2**	4-10 times	**6**
1-3 times	**4**	More than 10 times	**8**

12. I have normal weight. **3** I am seriously overweight (more than 20% above normal) **12**

    I am slightly overweight (up to 10% above normal) **6**

    I am moderately overweight (10-20% above normal) **9**

13. I seldom have illness or infections, and I recover or heal easily when I do. **1**

    I have occasional illness or infection, and I recover somewhat slowly. **3**

    I frequently am ill or have infections, and I heal slowly. **4**

14. My energy level is good and I recover from exertion easily. **1**

    I occasionally feel lethargic. **2**

    I tire very easily and need to rest frequently during the day. **4**

15. In the last year I have been hospitalized because my diabetes was out of control.

Never	**4**	More than once	**16**
Once	**9**		

B. Level of Regimen

These questions cover only the aspects of diabetes regimen that relate to metabolic control.

1. I am on an intensive insulin regimen (2 or more injections per day, using both regular and intermediate or long-acting insulin or the insulin pump) and vary dosage according to blood sugar tests. **3**

I take two injections per day but rarely vary dosage from
day to day.   **6**

I have only one injection of insulin each day.   **9**

NA   **6**

2. In the last two months I have forgotten or deliberately
    not taken insulin.

Never	**4**	More than twice	**16**
1-2 times	**12**	NA	**10.5**

3. I test blood glucose levels two or more times a day.   **3**

    I test blood glucose levels at least twice a week, or urine
    at least once a day.   **6**

    I test blood or urine at least twice a week.   **9**

    I seldom (or never) do any home urine or blood tests.   **12**

4. When my control is off (high or low blood sugar) or when
    there are changes in my routine (schedule, activity,
    food, or stress), I know how to alter insulin, diet, or
    activity to compensate for the changes. I can return
    to normal quickly.   **2**

    I make some general adjustments but sometimes
    don't get completely back to normal for a few days.   **4**

    I know when my control is off but rarely do
    anything to compensate.   **6**

    I don't know anything about adjusting insulin, food, or
    activity to maintain good control.   **8**

5. I measure or accurately estimate the amounts of food I
    eat and keep the prescribed balance of carbohydrate,
    protein, and fat.   **3**

    I usually eat in moderation and have a general awareness
    of the balance of carbohydrate, protein, and fat.   **6**

    I eat pretty much what I want to, but not to excess.   **9**

I frequently eat excessively or irregularly. **12**

6. I seldom eat sweets, and I minimize use of other simple carbohydrates (such as dried fruits and fruit juices). **3**

I eat small portions of sweets and other simple carbohydrates. **6**

I usually eat small portions, but at least once a week I binge. **9**

I eat all the sweets and fruit I want, sometimes a lot. **12**

7. I eat as little animal fat as possible (butter, fatty meat, luncheon meat, high fat cheese). **3**

I eat small amounts of animal fat and rarely eat excessive amounts. **6**

I usually eat only small amounts of animal fat, but at least once a week I eat a lot or binge. **9**

I eat all the animal fat I want. **12**

8. I eat complex carbohydrates and high fiber foods (whole grains, vegetables, etc.)

at most meals **2**

about half the time **4**

rarely **6**

never **8**

9. When I have overeaten or know that a large meal is coming, I use extra insulin or exercise to compensate for the extra calories

nearly always **2**

usually **4**

rarely **6**

never **8**

10. I have moderate to full physical activity regularly (the equivalent of 20 minutes of exercise with heart rate 120+). **2**

I have moderate physical activity, but it usually varies
quite a bit from day to day.   **4**

I am relatively inactive or irregular in my level of activity.   **6**

I am very inactive or very irregular in my level of activity.   **8**

11. When I am under emotional stress,

I feel able to cope well, and the stress does not seriously
affect my blood sugar level.   **2**

I try to cope, but my control may be off for the next few tests.   **4**

I don't cope too well, and my blood sugar level may be
high for a day or more.   **6**

I forget everything I know about coping, ignore my
diabetes, and my blood sugar stays high.   **8**

Add up the numbers you circled for parts A and B and enter your totals
here:

*Part A: Level of Control*_____

*Part B: Level of Regimen*_____

Now see what your level of control and level of management are.

Level of Control	Score	Level of Regimen	Score
Optimal	34-42	Intensive	28-42
Moderate	43-65	Moderate	43-63
Loose	66-90	Loose	64-84
Minimal	91+	Minimal	85+

These general ranges are derived from the authors' experience and
have been pilot tested, but they have not been fully validated. However, your score should give you a sense of where you are and what
you need to work on.

Completing this exercise can be challenging, maybe even downright
unpleasant. If your results were not as positive as you thought they
would be, don't blame yourself. Acknowledge the choices you have

been making and the reasons you have been making them. Give yourself room to begin making new choices. You might go through the regimen part of the questionnaire and check the places where you marked the higher numbers. These will indicate areas for needed improvement in management that you may feel willing to begin at this time. A little later in this chapter, there is another exercise that will help you choose the overall level of management you wish to exercise at this time.

In your answers to this questionnaire, you have a general profile of your current metabolic control regimen and your level of control. You may feel comfortable with this level of management, or other concerns may take priority. On the other hand, you may wish to improve control as your next step in living well with diabetes. You may wish to assume the intensive regimen. Or you may prefer to make the change in stages, working first to gain loose or moderate control.

BENEFITS OF ACHIEVING OPTIMAL CONTROL

The first thing you need to consider in choosing your level of diabetic regimen is what you can gain from the best level of control. You know achieving it will take effort. What will it give you?

Just beginning the learning process necessary to achieve optimal control often brings an immediate emotional benefit to many people with diabetes. We report a sense of greater power, less depression,and less anxiety. This emotional high helps us through the initial period of greater regulation required until we have learned the regimen. Once we have done so, we will experience greater freedom. We can deal with irregularities of diet, mealtimes, activity, and stress, and still obtain greatly improved blood sugar levels.

The first physical benefits start soon after control is improved. When blood sugar level is closer to normal, we simply feel better. We have more energy; we need to sleep less; we are less likely to grow fatigued. Our immune system works more effectively, so we are less likely to become ill or have infections that get out of control. When we do become seriously ill, we are better able to compensate for the effect of the physical stress on blood sugar, and we are less likely to develop ketoacidosis, a condition that can lead to diabetic coma. In formal studies, diabetics who maintained good control had many fewer hospitalizations, a considerable economic benefit.

Women who improve metabolic control develop fewer vaginal and urinary tract infections and consequently find greater enjoyment of sex. In addition, their menstrual periods become more regular. Adolescents are less likely to experience a delay in beginning menstruation. With strict control leading up to and continuing during pregnancy, the risks for both mother and child are greatly reduced. (In diabetes, very careful management of pregnancy is necessary. See Chapter 18, "Living Well As A Diabetic Woman.")

For children, optimal control encourages normal patterns of growth and development. (Growth is sometimes stunted when blood sugar is poorly controlled in childhood.) Fluctuations in insulin requirements caused by growth spurts and the hormonal changes during puberty are more easily handled with the intensive regimen. Parental awareness of the emotional side of diabetes can help children live well with the more demanding regimen.

These are the short-term benefits we can experience directly, but that's only half the story. Laboratory tests of diabetics in good control show that several important measures of physiological balance are brought to normal values. These include factors in the blood that are responsible for clotting; the levels of certain fats (cholesterol and triglycerides) that contribute to heat and circulatory disorders when they are high; the release of a variety of hormones; and even the thickness and fragility of capillaries (the thinnest blood vessels). All of these factors tend to be abnormal when blood sugar is high.

Although we don't experience symptoms from these abnormalities in the short run, their presence is not healthful. They are the basic building blocks from which diabetic complications are constructed over time. In the long run, high blood sugar levels increase the chance of developing heart disease, circulatory problems, blindness and other vision problems, kidney disorders, and neuropathy (nerve malfunctions).

These future possibilities support us in following a demanding regimen in the present. We work most effectively when this takes the form of healthy concern, not chronic anxiety.

Optimal control of diabetes has been possible for only a few years, not enough time to determine scientifically whether it will lower the chance of developing these long-term complications. But studies are now accumulating that document the effect of improved control in the short run. Capillary thickness, growth hormone levels, excessive fats in the blood, and factors affecting clotting have been normalized when blood sugar levels were brought under control. In this way, a major, but subtle, aspect of the *illness* of diabetes can be erased. We can live well with diabetes now and provide a basis for a future without major complications.

What if complications have already set in? Is it too late to bother with control? No, but discuss the cautions mentioned earlier in the chapter about cardiovascular disease, neuropathy, and kidney disease with your doctor. Even at this stage, one may benefit from improved control. In some cases, complications may be reversed or their impact lessened by careful management. Whether or not existing complications can be reversed, one's chances of avoiding or slowing the development of other complications are improved. The immediate physical benefits and the emotional lift gained by taking control help one deal more effectively with the fears that usually accompany the diagnosis of a complication. *(One additional caution: Control must be improved gradually if retinopathy or kidney disease at any stage has already started. See Chapter 17, "Complications Simplified," for details.)*

Optimal control of diabetes offers powerful benefits immediately and over the long run. But there is no guarantee that it will prevent future complications or reverse them once they have started. What it does do is improve our odds, reducing the risk of having complications. We feel that the decision to gain optimal control must be made in terms of the present benefits, which include having a body that functions more healthfully right now and that has less risk of developing complications later.

THE COSTS OF GAINING OPTIMAL CONTROL

What are the costs of better control? Economically, there is a moderate cost, one that more insurance companies are now covering. Blood test strips are still much more expensive that urine test materials, but there are ways of cutting corners (and the strips) to save money. At the time of most intensive testing (four to six times a day for the first weeks), the cost would be $15 to $25 a month by the economy route, but up to $100 a month without cutting costs. Some people choose to use a meter for reading the strips, at a cost of $50 to $200. With most meters, it is also necessary to use the full strip. The only other piece of equipment is an automatic fingerpicking device that lessens the chance of pain. It costs around $15.

During the first months of intensive control, there is a significant cost in time and energy. Collecting information, testing, keeping records, figuring out what the records mean—all this becomes a major project. But probably it is no more complex than learning to drive. Depending on how much new information you have to acquire, the task could take anywhere from three to ten hours a week.

Another cost at the beginning: You need to regularize all aspects of life that affect blood sugar, making changes that may or may not be simple. The more you do this, the more quickly you will reach the point where you do not have to be so regular. It is much easier to learn how to keep your blood sugar within limits if you follow fairly set routines during the training period. Without this regularity, it is difficult to know what is causing tests to be too high or too low. Once you know the ropes, you'll enjoy much more freedom.

One potential liability when maintaining strict control: You are likely to have more insulin reactions. This is especially true if you have usually had high blood sugar levels or have been irregular in activity or diet. (Often, fear of reactions is one of the reasons a person with diabetes will keep blood sugar high.) Meanwhile, you will need to sharpen awareness of the cues indicating that a reaction is on its way and be sure to always have some form of sugar with you. With home blood testing, you can easily check whether those "funny feelings" are the result of low blood sugar or some other cause, like anxiety. "Hypoglycemic unawareness" is being recognized more often, and researchers are studying the causes.

Testing is especially important if you find that your reaction symptoms have become more subtle. Some people experience a decrease in the output of stress hormones that signal the appearance of an insulin reaction. They also exhaust the glycogen (sugar reserves) stored in the liver. When this develops, blood sugar can drop quite low without triggering the usual alarms—shakiness, sweating, increased pulse rate, and so forth. If you feel it has become difficult to tell when an insulin reaction is occurring, talk with your doctor. It is an important consideration when determining the level of control you will try to maintain. Although hypoglycemic unawareness used to be considered a form of diabetic nerve disease that developed in people with diabetes for many years, it is now realized that this can also happen early in diabetes.

We have included in the following pages many safeguards against insulin reactions. In Chapter 8, we give comprehensive information on reactions, including tips on recognizing and treating them.

Weighing the Costs and Benefits

Take a moment to consider how these benefits and costs of optimal control balance out for you.

- What value do you place on the benefits we have described?

  _____

- Which are the most important to you?

  _____

- Do any of the costs seem particularly heavy to you?

  _____

- If so, what could you do to lighten them?

  _____

A CHOICE OF REGIMEN

Given the benefits of optimal control, one might conclude that the treatment plan designed to bring it about should be the only one offered to people with diabetes. This would be a profound mistake. We cannot ignore the obvious fact that diabetes care is just one of the many items we must manage in our lives. Until the next set of technical breakthroughs, optimal control will depend on a set of life-style changes and an educational process requiring time and intense effort. Those of us who are not prepared to make these changes or those with extraordinary demands on time and energy might choose to ignore our diabetes if we feel we cannot follow the optimal path.

Therefore, it makes more sense to offer a choice of alternative regimens—*a continuum of self-care*. This choice, made consciously or subconsciously, is reflected in our day-to-day actions. And there is an infinite range of actions along the continuum from intensive to loose. We do what we do, with or without the knowledge and support of our physician or health care team. It makes sense to recognize this and support each person in the choices made. With this approach, you can begin at the level where you feel willing to work and proceed at a pace that is right for you.

The Intensive Regimen

The first choice we will consider is the regimen that allows you to gain nearly normal blood sugar values in a few months. This optimal control of diabetes depends upon a number of innovations in self-care, knit together into a state-of-the-art management program. We call this the intensive regimen.

The Intensive Regimen

1. Home blood sugar testing (blood glucose monitoring) two to four times a day (as many as six times a day at the beginning).

2. Insulin injections two to four times a day, usually using both rapid-acting and intermediate or long-acting insulins, or continuous insulin delivery by insulin pump.

3. Knowledge of food values and ability to follow a diet that ensures normal body weight, diabetic control, and reduced risk of complications.

4. An active life style, an exercise program, or both, followed regularly.

5. Ability to alter insulin dosage, food intake, and activity level to compensate for irregularities and the effects of stress.

6. Knowledge of the role of physical and emotional stress in diabetes and the ability to manage both.

7. Commitment to continuing diabetes learning, maintaining motivation, and meeting one's emotional needs.

The old staples of diabetes care are all here—insulin, diet, exercise—but we've added several new ingredients. In this approach, home blood glucose monitoring allows precise feedback about blood sugar level, information that enables you to make more precise decisions about insulin dosage, activity, and diet. When you test your blood several times a day, multiple injections or the pump can provide a pattern of insulin action closely matching the peaks of blood sugar following meals.

Awareness of the effect of stress on diabetic control helps you understand many puzzling swings in blood sugar levels. More effective management of stressful situations helps to reduce the metabolic effect of these swings. Furthermore, the intensive regimen recognizes that the demands of the regimen itself may become a source of stress. So it includes work to make these demands less burdensome and to help you stay motivated. For the regimen to work in the long run, it must serve as a foundation for the rest of your life, not as a substitute for living.

Who Needs the Intensive Regimen?

Some people will choose this path simply because they tend to do their best in everything they do or because they have strong motivation to live as heathfully as possible. However, others will make this choice because of a specific and immediate health need.

The intensive regimen is especially recommended for

- Women who are pregnant or are planning to become pregnant.

- Patients with diabetic complications beginning to develop (nerve and kidney disorders, circulatory problems, heart disease, retinopathy, and other eye disorders). (If retinopathy or kidney disease has started, you may need to proceed gradually. See Chapter 17, "Complications Simplified.")

- Children whose growth is significantly behind schedule.

- Patients with other chronic illnesses or conditions, where the consequences of high blood sugar make the other chronic conditions worse.

People in these categories often choose to make optimal control a high priority and to reorder other aspects of their lives that might interfere. If personal obstacles are making it hard for you to make this level of commitment, you may wish to seek assistance in the form of individual counseling or a support group. If you decide to continue with a moderate or loose regimen because other problems are more pressing, you can review your decision periodically to see if a new choice seems possible.

You may need to adopt a somewhat less strict version of the intensive regimen if you have difficulty recognizing the symptoms of an insulin reaction. After many years of diabetes, the usual signs of low blood sugar sometimes diminish or disappear because of hormonal changes. Your doctor can order tests to determine whether this has happened to you. If your hormonal output is normal, then you need to sharpen your awareness of the physical cues of low blood sugar. Medicines for some other conditions (typically beta blockers for high blood pressure) can also blunt your recognition of symptoms.

The Moderate Regimen

If we discussed only the intensive regimen, some of you, unable or unwilling to devote yourself to diabetes care in such a concentrated fashion, would be left out in the cold. If you are facing extraordinary demands, if you have little motivation or a highly individualistic style, or if you have any emotional obstacles, you may need a regimen that respects your particular needs: a slower, less concentrated pace; a freer structure allowing you more room for dealing with your concerns; and a periodic review of your choice of regimen. It is possible to include in the moderate regimen many innovations of the intensive regimen so that you can significantly improve your control, since we are talking about a continuum of self-care, not an all-or-none situation.

The Moderate Regimen

1. Regular home blood glucose testing (at least two or four times a week, best daily, and as needed) combined with daily urine tests.

2. One or two insulin injections daily, usually with a combination of rapid-acting and intermediate or long-acting insulins. (The insulin pump is not recommended with this regimen.)

3. Knowledge of food values and ability to follow a diet that ensures normal body weight and moderate diabetic control.

4. An active life style, a regular exercise program, or both.

5. Ability to make cautious adjustments in insulin dosage, food intake, and activity level to compensate for changes and the effects of stress.

6. Knowledge of the role of physical and emotional stress in diabetes and the ability to manage either.

7. Commitment to continuing diabetes learning, maintaining motivation, and meeting your own emotional needs.

The moderate regimen differs from the intensive regimen in the level of feedback and control it provides. Testing is less rigorous and, as a result, the style of insulin dosage cannot be so finely tailored. Without frequent blood tests, you have too little information to make precise daily adjustments in insulin dosage, food, or activity. Caution is recommended. For this reason, the insulin pump or more than two insulin injections a day are not recommended for anyone on either the moderate or the loose regimen.

Home blood sugar testing is an important part of the moderate regimen, even when it is done only a few times a week. The accuracy of the results, compared with urine tests, helps to build motivation to improve control. Having the strips on hand means that you can easily see how stress, a large meal, or an unusual level of exercise affects blood sugar. When you are ill, you can handle blood sugar and ketone problems more accurately. If you have difficulty detecting insulin reactions, you can use the tests to confirm hypoglycemia and to help develop more awareness of symptoms.

Sometimes, success in improving control has the unexpected effect of increasing your motivation dramatically. If you feel now that you could never handle the intensive regimen, you may find that the act of beginning to improve management gives you greater willingness later. Whether or not this occurs, you will feel much better about yourself than if you just continued in your old ways, believing that you could not control your diabetes. You will be dealing with one of the most important issues in your life—living well with diabetes.

The Loose Regimen

For those of you who may feel that even the moderate regimen is too restrictive or too demanding, you have a third choice. In the loose regimen, the focus is on identifying whatever you are willing to do to start improving control, and then doing it. In this regimen, we emphasize building willingness and a positive attitude, even though you may be living with a low level of control now. One important element for many diabetics who maintain this level is to face the fact that loose control is a choice they have made consciously or unconsciously. It is not something that just happens to them. It is useful to define this as a level of regimen rather than as a rebellion against or neglect of regimen. Both authors have managed their diabetes at this level in the past. Each of us has the right to choose how we live with our bodies. Learning to accept the choices we make helps us move on to more healthful choices.

The Loose Regimen

1. Knowledge of blood testing techniques, even though tests may be done infrequently. Urine testing several times a week.

2. One or two insulin injections daily. (More injections or the insulin pump are not recommended without regular blood sugar testing.)

3. Eating a healthful diet, usually in moderation.

4. Caution in adjusting insulin dosage, food intake, and activity level.

5. Commitment to continuing diabetes learning, maintaining motivation, and reviewing obstacles to improving control.

You may choose the loose regimen because your attention is focused on other areas in your life. If you do choose this level, remember that the time you do give to improving your diabetes management will probably help you manage the rest of your life better.

CHOOSING YOUR REGIMEN LEVEL

If you still have not decided which level of regimen to follow, answering these questions may help you to do so.

1. I need to achieve improved control soon because

_____ I have diabetic complications.

_____ I am pregnant.

_____ I am planning to become pregnant.

_____ I am a child whose growth is significantly below normal.

_____ I have another major illness.

2. I should be cautious about initiating an intensive regimen because
   _____ I do not experience the usual symptoms of low blood sugar and it is difficult for me to detect insulin reactions.

   _____ I have significant kidney, cerebrovascular, or cardiovascular disease.

   _____ I have beginning diabetic retinopathy or nephropathy.

3. The reasons I have for wishing to improve my control of diabetes include_____
   _____

4. a. Other major problems that need my attention now are_____
   _____

   b. I could gain assistance and support in dealing with these issues by _____

   c. Could I postpone working on any of these to gain time for diabetes? _____

5. The external support I now have for dealing with diabetes is
   _____abundant

   _____adequate

   _____inadequate

6. In making this decision, I also have to consider _____
   _____

Review your answers, discuss them with your physician and people close to you, and then make a decision you are happy with.

7. Given the above, my choice of regimen is

   intensive _____ moderate _____ loose _____ .

```
C  H  A  P  T  E  R      5
```

The Intensive Regimen

You learn much more easily when you divide large projects into manageable steps. You can see each task more clearly, and you can see the progress you make toward your overall goal. This definition of steps is doubly important when the project is learning the intensive regimen and making significant changes in life-style. The sequence in which you learn can make the enterprise safer and quicker. You may already have some of the required skills or knowledge, but we urge you to review all of the information we provide in this book. You may learn some facts you haven't seen elsewhere.

Eleven Steps to Optimal Control

1. Create a positive foundation. Be sure you have a positive setting for learning the intensive regimen, a physician who agrees with your goals, and support from family, friends, and other people with diabetes.

   Review the tools available to help you if you become frustrated or discouraged along the way. (See Chapters 3 and 14.)

2. Under your doctor's supervision, have lab tests of hemoglobin A$_1$c and blood lipids (triglycerides and cholesterol) done to indicate your present level of control.

   This gives you a benchmark with which to measure the effect of your new regimen.

3. Learn the skills and information basic to the intensive regimen:

   a. Learn how to test blood sugar and urine.
      The criteria of diabetic control.
      An effective record-keeping system.
      The meaning of each laboratory test relevant to diabetic control.

   b. Review Chapter 8, "Living Well With Insulin Reactions." It is important to review this because you may experience different signs of reaction when your metabolism is under better control, as well as more frequent reactions.

   c. Survey the basics of diabetic metabolism (how your system processes food and liquids to produce energy).

   d. Understand all of the different factors that determine blood sugar level.

4. Regularize diet and activity or exercise as much as possible during this period of learning. Later on you will have greater freedom.

5. Begin the period of intensive testing and record keeping without making any changes in regimen (unless your doctor requests changes). Keep careful records, and observe how you respond to your present regimen.

6. With your doctor's guidance, select the intensive insulin regimen best suited to you (two or more shots a day or the insulin pump). Begin this regimen and make the adjustments in it needed to obtain the best possible level of control.

7. Observe the variations in blood sugar level caused by stress, illness, changes in food and exercise, and other factors.

   a. Learn to vary insulin dosage, diet and exercise to compensate for high or low tests and to deal with changes in routine.

8. Have new lab tests done after two to three months to determine the effect of your new regimen and to establish your ongoing regimen.

9. Assess your progress and determine what, if anything, is needed to further improve control.

10. Take steps to maintain your motivation for continuing at this level of management.

11. Celebrate!

Step 1: Create a positive foundation

You are starting one of the most positive and challenging things you can do for yourself as a person with diabetes. The rewards at physical and emotional levels are profound. You may have to overcome many obstacles to gain these rewards. So your first step is making sure that the foundation for this work is also positive. This includes creating realistic expectations, neutralizing past failures at improving diabetes management, lining up professional and personal support, and becoming familiar with the things you can do if progress grinds to a halt.

One of the most useful expectations to have about this process is that it will take time. You can't just flip a switch and gain instant control. People who are willing and able to focus energy on gaining control quickly will find that the process takes one to two months and sometimes longer. It is possible to meet with repeated discouragement, even when committing to an all-out effort. This is particularly true for people with physiological problems such as partial immunity to insulin, and those with a high level of emotional or environmental stress. These people may follow the diabetic regimen perfectly and gain improved control, but still experience large fluctuations in blood sugar level.

If at first you don't succeed, find out what else you need to do. Discuss what is happening with your doctor or diabetes educator, be patient with yourself and keep giving yourself credit for what you have achieved. Sometimes improving diabetic control calls for a prescription of a stress management class, couples counseling, or transfer to a less stressful job. Or a more highly purified insulin may be needed to overcome immunity that can develop after years of injections.

Occasionally, it becomes necessary to accept a lesser degree of control than you would like to have because, at the time, you are unwilling to make the changes called for. If so, spare yourself the additional stress of feeling guilty. Respect your decision and keep the postponed changes on your agenda.

We discussed in the Introduction ways to safeguard against failure. There is probably no more important place to apply them than when learning the intensive regimen. If you start down this path and then feel you are failing, it is time to use Chapters 3 and 14, the "Help!" and "Living Well With Yourself" chapters, designed to help you overcome the obstacles you have encountered. You are not really failing; you just have something else to learn before you can succeed. Although you may feel a sense of urgency about the learning, it is helpful to drop your judgments. Transform obstacles into a natural part of the learning process, letting them define the next lessons you must master.

Those of us who have tried many times to improve our metabolic control may have to set aside a history of frustration and lack of success. In the past, we simply did not have adequate tools to achieve our goal. Now, it is important to let go of that old feeling, "I'll never get this right." It is time for a completely fresh effort.

The fear and sense of urgency that inspire many who decide to learn the intensive regimen need to be balanced with more positive motivation. Fear is a powerful feeling. It can move us for a time, but our progress is steadier and more enduring when it is grounded in a positive sense of oneself—in our basic wellness.

Ernest's Experience

I'm afraid I have to confess, I didn't really start to take control of diabetes until the ophthalmologist told me I had a high risk of going blind. I learned fast then. I enjoy the world's beauty too much to lose my vision of it.

But soon I realized that everything I was doing was for all of me, not just to save my eyes. I was giving myself a degree of love and respect that I'd always withheld before.

After a few months, I had the first hemorrhage in my left eye. And then, after laser treatment, another, and yet another. I could see only a blur through that eye. I had to face the strong possibility of losing vision in both eyes. When the difficulties started, I half expected to give up on my intensive regimen with the childish feeling, "It didn't do any good, anyway." Why didn't I? It's simple: I feel better loving and respecting myself, no matter what the outcome of my actions may be. I am living well, despite the possibility of losing my sight.

As I'm writing, I'm watching cows swishing their tails in the shade of a large oak, against golden hills. Above my keyboard there's a lovely bronze statue of Krishna, a flute-playing god who herds cows in Indian mythology. Once, when I asked my eye doctor what he thought would happen with my eyes, he answered with an unconscious pun, "We'll just have to wait and see." I replied, "I certainly hope so." I waited, and I'm seeing. The laser treatment was successful.

Eleven years after laser treatment I am pleased to tell you that I have not had a hemorrhage for four years. There are very small leaks of blood that give me more floaters than most people my age. But I see this beautiful· world—the trees I plant, the flowers I grow, and that statue of Krishna—with 20/20 vision.

Another important part of this first step is reviewing and strengthening your support system. A key element is, of course, your physician. You need one who is well informed about the newer approaches to diabetes care and who endorses your increased role in managing your condition. Discuss what you are doing thoroughly with your doctor and work out ground rules for the management decisions you are to make at each step. Most physicians are very pleased when they see their patients taking greater responsibility, and they support their independence fully. Often they make it possible for you to discuss test results and special problems by phone between office visits and provide twenty-four hour access in case of emergencies. Ask about this if your doctor doesn't suggest it.

The encouragement of your family can help a great deal during that time. Let the people close to you know what you are working on and what it means to you. Share your concerns and expectations. Ask for the help you need or for changes in any family patterns that interfere with your efforts to improve management. If you are in a negative family situation, you may need to take action to neutralize your family's influence and look for more support from others.

You should also let your friends know about your project and ask them for assistance. This can be very helpful when you are attempting to make basic life style changes. Friendships often revolve around habitual behavior and may be threatened when you start changing habits. You can reduce the threat and gain valuable aid if you communicate the importance of the changes you are making. Realize, though, that some friends may be too attached to their old image of you. If they offer little support, let that be their problem, not yours.

Support from other diabetics, especially those who are also learning the intensive regimen, is second only to guidance of your physician during this period. Individual contacts or a support group can offer excellent encouragement and reinforcement, as well as sharing of practical tips on many details of management. Some physicians even organize a buddy system or support group for people working on improving control. Such groups could be organized by a few individuals working through their local American Diabetes Association chapter, or on their own, if necessary.

The last task in this initial phase is remembering the support and guidance you can give yourself when you feel stuck, frustrated, confused, blocked, or otherwise discouraged. Chances are very good that you will reach this point one or two times in the coming months. It is a natural part of the process. Now, when you are still full of enthusiasm, is a good time to plant the seeds for the times when you may forget how creative you are. Glance through "Help!" and "Living Well With Yourself" (Chapters 3 and 14). Review your strengths and skills. You might even write a note to yourself to be opened when you feel that you can't go on. Remind yourself of all the things you can do at a time when you feel there is nothing you can do.

Summary of Step 1

Begin by creating a positive foundation for the work of learning the intensive regimen. Review your support system and strengthen it where it is weak. This includes support from yourself as well as from your doctor, family, friends, and other diabetics. Remember that this is a fail-safe process designed to help you overcome any obstacles that may arise.

Step 2: Have laboratory tests done to provide a benchmark of control

Discuss with your physician the tests that will provide an accurate indication of your present level of control. The ones usually used include hemoglobin A_1c, fasting or random glucose, and blood lipids (the fats, triglycerides, and cholesterol). (These are described in Step 3). The results of these tests, along with your other records, tell you how far you have to go to obtain optimal control. But, more important, they will tell you how far you have come after a few weeks of learning. The objective feedback you receive when you compare the next set of lab tests with these may be very encouraging. Or, if there is little improvement, the new tests (together with your records of home tests, diet, stress, and exercise) will help you determine what to do next.

Step 3: Learn the skills and information basic to the intensive regimen

3a. Learn How to Test Blood Sugar and Urine.

Learn how to test your own blood for glucose (the type of sugar predominant in human blood), the relationship of this test to urine tests, the meaning of the different laboratory tests your physician requests, and a record-keeping method that makes it easy to monitor your day-to-day control.

Self blood glucose testing is possibly the greatest advance in diabetes care since the discovery of insulin. It is a powerful feedback system that gives accurate information about the level of your blood sugar. On the basis of these data, you can make decisions regarding precise insulin dosage, exercise, diet, stress, and reactions. It is one of the keys you can use to achieve both optimal metabolic control and greater freedom in your life.

You can understand the importance of this tool if you consider the automatic "testing" process in a person who does not have diabetes. There is a continuous, unconscious monitoring of blood sugar level, with feedback to the pancreas and other organs releasing hormones that maintain a normal level. The control information is available within seconds; insulin and other hormones regulating blood sugar level begin acting immediately. When the blood sugar level rises after a meal, the pancreas releases insulin into the bloodstream. If the nondiabetic feels under attack or if blood sugar falls because of exercise, glucose is released by the liver, and adrenalin and other hormones inhibit the action of insulin. Through these processes, blood glucose levels are kept between 60 and 120 in the nondiabetic.

As you know, when you developed type I diabetes, you lost all or part of your ability to produce insulin. You still generate the other hormones that cause blood sugar to rise and fall, but the key hormone that allows cells to utilize blood sugar is missing. The inner testing signals high blood sugar, but there is little or no response from the pancreas.

So you have to enter into the control process consciously, injecting insulin and monitoring blood sugar level by tests and by how you feel. Your feelings tell you when your blood sugar level is too low and you are having an insulin reaction; and they tell you when you have very high blood sugar. But you cannot feel the difference between normal (70-120 mg/dl), slightly high (121-180 mg/dl), and moderately high (181-240 mg/dl) levels. Until the last dozen years, the only day-to-day tests were urine glucose sticks or tablets that give only a rough idea of blood sugar level. They do not give up-to-the-minute feedback; they only indicate whether you are a little out of control or very out of control. They do have their use in diabetes care, but it is limited.

Self blood glucose testing, on the other hand, gives information on your level of control at the time of the test. You can get a relatively accurate reading (within 10 to 20% of the actual value) in the critical area where urine tests only read "negative"' (below 180 mg/dl). With this feedback, you can tell when you need extra insulin (or less food) and how much. You know when you are having an insulin reaction and you do not mistake the symptoms of an anxiety attack for those of low blood sugar. You know the precise effect on blood sugar level of a particular meal or snack or of a period of exercise. By making conscious decisions about all of this information, you can guide your body to a level of metabolic control that is more nearly normal.

This precise feedback of blood sugar level has a strong impact on the behavior of most diabetics who do blood testing. It becomes easier to deal with the craving for a hot fudge sundae when you've seen your blood sugar shoot up to 450 mg/dl upon eating one. That much-postponed stress management class becomes a high priority when you've seen a distressing day at work produce a record high in blood sugar. With home blood glucose testing, you have a tool for understanding in detail exactly how you live with diabetes. You start to understand the reasons for the highs and lows, and you gain increasing ability to do something about them. That's living well!

Supplies You Will Need for Self Blood Glucose Testing

- Blood glucose testing reagent strips: Appropriate strips for visual reading or the strips used in the blood glucose meter you use.

- Lancets: Monolet by Monoject Division of Sherwood Medical (or other manufacturers), or the needle of a disposable syringe.

- Alcohol and cotton balls or tissue.

- An easy-to-read watch with a second hand or timer (if you don't use a meter, see below).

- (Optional) A small device that pricks fingers automatically. Monoject makes one called the Autolet, Bio-Dynamics makes the Autoclix, and Palco makes the Auto-Lancet. Several others are also available.

- A meter for reading the strips is advisable for many people. Ones that "speak" the blood sugar reading are now available for people with impaired vision. Mail-order diabetes supply centers sell them at a discount. (See Appendix.)

Testing equipment and supplies may be covered by your health insurance.

Using a blood glucose meter gives more exact results than can be obtained from visually reading Chemstrips or Visidex strips. For this reason, pregnant women and those using the insulin pump should use meters. People with color blindness or other visual impairment need them as well. Anyone fascinated with gadgetry may find that the little machine boosts their motivation to test.

Since a variety of strips and meters are available, and new ones keep appearing, we will not give specific testing instructions here. The new meters are very user-friendly, even smaller and much more automatic than the old meters. We encourage you to attend a class in blood glucose testing at a diabetes clinic or to have your procedures and interpretation checked by your physician or nurse. Frequently, training is provided by the meter vendor. We will, however, offer some tips and cautions that will help you with your home blood testing.

To ensure the accuracy of your readings, test in a space that is at least 60 degrees F, or breathe gently on the strip while the blood is on it to keep it warm. Use the side of your fingertips, which is less painful. Never use so small a drop of blood that you have to smear it on the strip (the blood should stay liquid during the testing time). Never use gauze to remove the blood (it may scrape off the test material). If timing is not automatic, keep your timing to within three to five seconds of the required time (don't estimate). Never use test strips after they have expired.

If you visually read the test strips, be sure to estimate blood sugar level when the colors fall between the ones on the container. A chief source of error is automatically choosing one of the "official" scores when the colors are actually midway between the colors given. Do not match your test strip with a color chart other than the one on the container in which it came.

Here are a few of the objections and concerns about home blood testing that are raised by users.

"I'm afraid it'll hurt." We already stick ourselves at least once a day to take insulin, yet fingertips seem more sensitive, somehow, than thighs and upper arms. Actually, there is usually little pain, especially along the sides of the fingertips. Often you hardly feel the prick. With

the automatic devices adjusted to the proper depth, you almost never notice when the lancet strikes. The anticipation of the pain is far worse than anything you actually experience. Also, your fingertips do not become sore or tender from repeated pricks. (It is a good idea to rotate from finger to finger, just as insulin shots are given in a different site each time.)

Actively in development are "non-invasive" meters that will read your blood sugar through the skin, without requiring a drop of blood. Rumors are that they will be quite expensive, at least initially.

"Won't it be terribly expensive if I start testing several times a day?" Costs can be cut in two ways. With visually read tests, you can cut the strips lengthwise in two with scissors. If you have sharp eyes, you can cut them into three or four strips, once you have learned to interpret the readings accurately. (Be sure to put unused strips back into the container right away. Cut strips have been tested and found to give reliable results, even when stored cut for a month. Some meters allow for using a half strip, but with most you must use a whole one.)

Second, you can buy the strips from a discount mail-order firm (see Appendix). At the time of this writing, each test costs about 12 cents if discounted strips are cut four ways. Uncut, the cost of each strip is 48 cents. If you have health insurance, check to see if it covers testing equipment and supplies. More and more medical plans are covering these costs.

"Won't I get discouraged if I see too many high tests?" Probably you will, and you can deal with the discouragement by remembering that this is only one of several steps in learning to control your blood sugar. High tests indicate only that you have more to learn, not that you are weak or unable to learn. You can use these tests to increase your motivation to master the regimen.

"Can children handle home blood testing?" Children can do it, with the proper support and guidance of adults. (It helps if the adults stick their own fingers and test their own blood a few times to offer encouragement and a good example.) Four- and five-year-olds have learned the testing procedure, though usually they are a few years older before they start doing their own tests. In fact, once they are trained in testing, children become excellent instructors of their peers.

"How often do I have to test?" Curiosity may lead you to do fairly frequent testing at first. It is very satisfying to be able to determine the exact impact of a given food, activity, or stress on your blood sugar level. For the first month or two of the intensive regimen, you may need to test up to six times a day to get a clear picture of your pattern of response. This would include tests before each meal, at bedtime, and, at least part of the time, one or two hours after a meal.

"I can tell by how I feel whether I'm high or low." This is true only if you are very high or very low. Usually, you cannot sense much without actual symptoms. You may be able to learn to sense blood sugar level in the midrange (70-200 mg/dl) by using the feedback from your blood tests. You might try jotting down your guesstimate before testing for a few weeks. Write down the level you think you are at (given what you know about what you have eaten and done since the last test), and also write down the first number that pops into your mind. See if you come close to your actual test using either method.

Interpreting Blood Glucose Tests

With optimal control of diabetes, the test values you attain can be close to the blood sugar levels of a person who does not have diabetes. The following table gives the target glucose levels recommended by Jay Skyler, one of the leading diabetologists in the United States.

Intensive Regimen Target Glucose Levels

Time	Ideal	Acceptable Level
Fasting	60-90 mg/dl	60-105 mg/dl
Before meal	60-105 mg/dl	60-130 mg/dl
1 hr after meal	140 mg/dl or less	180 mg/dl or less
2 hr after meal	120 mg/dl or less	150 mg/dl or less

These are demanding standards, requiring full practice of the intensive regimen. If you can achieve them, fine. If not, keep working to improve your control. And remember that you are acceptable even when your test results are not. You and your doctor may agree on a higher set of target levels to begin with if these seem too difficult to attain. Or you may have to shift your targets up if you have too many insulin reactions.

By checking your blood sugar one to two hours after a meal, you will begin to learn how the food you have just eaten is affecting your sugar level. This information will greatly refine your skill in using your intuition, symptoms, general feelings, and blood tests to predict how different foods will affect your control. Knowing this, you will be in a better position to choose the target blood sugar levels appropriate for you.

Urine Testing

In the intensive regimen, urine testing is still very useful for checking for ketones in the urine. You should keep ketone test supplies on hand, especially for when you are ill or stressed. Both tablets and strips are available. (A new home blood test strip is now available for testing ketones, called KetoSite. It is manufactured by GDS Diagnostics, Elkhart, Indiana.)

The traditional test for sugar in the urine is useful chiefly in the moderate and loose regimens. For anyone on the intensive regimen, the test does not offer the precise feedback needed to maintain optimal control. For this reason, it is covered in the section on the moderate regimen.

Metabolic Record Keeping

Keeping clear records that you and your doctor can learn from is as important as doing the testing itself. At the beginning, we recommend that you log your tests, diet, activity level, and stress. (Once control is established, less detailed records will be sufficient.) During this initial period, you are a scientist studying your own metabolism. The information you gather will help you learn more quickly about your individual patterns of response.

Here are forms you can photocopy for a daily log and for a periodic summary of your records. For the daily log, you can choose between a simple form that allows you to see the pattern of test results easily but that does not allow detailed recording of food and activity, and a more elaborate one that provides space for more detailed record keeping. (See page 120 for examples of filled-in logs in Step 7 below.) Some meters now have memories to record test results. They can also be hooked to computers for printouts and analyses.

Daily Diabetes Log I

DATE TIME	INSULIN DOSE	BREAK-FAST TEST	LUNCH TEST	DINNER TEST	BED TEST	COMMENTS: Illness, change of pattern, stress

Daily Diabetes Log II

DATE TIME	BLOOD TEST & REACTIONS	INSULIN DOSAGE	ACTIVITY & EXERCISE	FOOD	COMMENTS: Stress, illness, etc.

When you miss a test, indicate your estimate: "est. high" or "est. 150." Include reactions in the blood sugar test column, with the amount of food used to treat it in the food column. Grade reactions as mild (1), strong (2), or severe (3). Indicate the type of insulin if more than one type is used.

Grade activity for each period of the day relative to what is normal for you at that time: 1 = minimal activity, 2 = less activity than usual, 3 = your normal level, 4 = more activity than usual, 5 = maximum activity. Include length of time of activity or exercise.

Under "Food," indicate calories or exchanges and anything out of the ordinary, such as delayed meals. If you calculate only carbohydrates, indicate over- or underconsumption. You may wish to note the particular foods consumed.

Under "Comments," include any stressful events, whether or not you sensed having an emotional response. Note difficulty with sleeping, times of special tension or relaxation, good feelings, and any physical occurrences such as illness, the beginning of menstruation, low energy—anything that might help to explain the variations in your tests.

Remember, these records are not just for your doctor. Useful as they are to your physician, they are even more valuable to you. Analyze them, learn from them, and make changes based on what you learn from them. By writing down this information, you give yourself a tool for seeing the patterns of your life with diabetes. (The interpretation of these records is discussed in Step 7.)

Lab Tests Your Physician May Order

When you are testing your own blood sugar regularly at home, the traditional fasting blood glucose test at the lab becomes less important. It can give you a quality check on your testing technique. (Bring your testing materials and do your own test at the same time your blood is drawn at the lab.) If there is a significant difference (more than 10%), ask your doctor or nurse to review your procedure.

The lab is able to make other important tests with the same sample of blood. A relatively new one, hemoglobin A_1c (or glycosylated hemoglobin), gives an overall evaluation of blood sugar control. This test measures the amount of glucose that has bound to the hemoglobin in the red blood cells. Since the average blood cell lasts for two to three months, the test results give an approximate summary or average of your blood sugar levels over that period. Higher readings usually indicate need for a change in regimen or in your level of adherence.

Hemoglobin A₁c and Control

4.0-8.0	Normal in nondiabetics
Less than 8.0	Good control of diabetes
8.0-10	Fair control
More than 10	Poor control

(Slightly different test methods are used in each lab, so different values may be used to evaluate your test. Ask your doctor or the lab technician for those being used in your test.)

A home test for hemoglobin A_1c is now available so you can test yourself between lab visits. It is called Self Assure GHb and can be obtained from the diabetic discount supply houses listed at the end of this book. A new lab test, not yet widely accepted or available, gives a measure for average blood glucose level over a three-week period. It's called a fructosamine assay and is marketed under the name RoTag. Check with your doctor.

Another set of blood tests reflects overall control. These tests measure certain blood fats (or lipids). High levels of cholesterol or triglycerides are commonly associated with high blood sugar values in diabetes. Their presence over long periods contributes to the development of diabetic complications. These blood lipids should be tested every year or two if they are in the normal range. If your tests are high and you are working to reduce them with diet and control, it is helpful to have the tests done every two or three months. It is also useful to measure high-density lipoprotein cholesterol (HDLC), the "good" cholesterol (the more you have, the better).

Normal Values for Blood Lipids

The National Institutes of Health Expert Adult Treatment Panel has made simplified recommendations on cholesterol and triglyceride levels. (Formerly they were determined according to age and sex.)

Total cholesterol below 200 mg/dl is considered desirable; between 200 and 240, borderline high; and greater than 240, high.

Those with levels over 240 should have their low-density lipoprotein (LDL) and HDL cholesterols and triglycerides measured, although some believe anyone with diabetes should have HDL, LDL, and triglycerides measured, irrespective of the level of total cholesterol. LDL levels of 160 mg/dl or greater are considered high risk; 130-159, borderline high risk; and less than 130, desirable. Although desired HDL levels are somewhat controversial, levels less than 35 mg/dl are considered a risk factor, and those greater than 60 are considered protective. Rather than looking at absolute levels of HDL, others consider the ratio of total cholesterol to HDL cholesterol a better measure of risk: The higher the HDL, the lower (and more desirable) the ratio, with ratios of 3.5-4 to 1 considered satisfactory. Triglycerides should probably be less than 250 mg/dl and treated with medication if greater than 500.

CAUTION: All of these numbers are subject to your specific situation, and how they apply to you should be discussed with your physician.

Tests and Our Emotions

It is natural to feel discouraged, and perhaps even guilty, when home or lab tests show that you are not in very good control. If the tests are high enough, you may despair and feel like throwing in the towel. At times like this, it is important to remember that you don't have to feel guilty about your errors and limitations. Use them to guide your next steps of learning. The energy of discouragement and guilt can be recycled into new motivation for change.

3b. Learn How to Recognize and Treat Insulin Reactions

This step is so important that we have given it a whole chapter, a chapter you should read even if you've had diabetes for years and think you know everything there is to know about insulin reactions. The symptoms of reactions change, becoming more subtle, when our metabolism is well controlled. Since our blood sugar is closer to normal, irregularities in food, activity, or schedule may cause reactions to occur more frequently at first.

In addition, some of us find it difficult to recognize the symptoms of a reaction. Sometimes this is because of changes in the output of hormones that signal low blood sugar. Review Chapter 8 for information on these subjects and other new ideas on increasing awareness of the early symptoms of a reaction and ensuring that you wake up to nighttime hypoglycemia.

3c. Survey the Basics of Diabetic Metabolism

Diabetes is a disorder of metabolism, the complex set of processes through which the food we eat becomes energy and replenishes our tissues. When we have diabetes, we play an active role in these processes, guiding things that happen automatically in nondiabetics. So we need to learn about our metabolism, especially as it relates to blood glucose.

Let's begin with some praise for blood glucose. We spend so much time trying to control it that we may forget how vital it is to our lives. Glucose is a major fuel for all of our cells and the only source of energy for the brain and nerve tissue. We have direct experience of this important function in the confusion we sometimes experience with an insulin reaction; it is a sign that not enough glucose is reaching the brain. We can respect our blood glucose, even as we work to keep it within acceptable limits.

The carbohydrates we eat are the main source of blood glucose. The different forms of starch and sugar in fruits and vegetables, beans and grains, and dairy foods are all transformed into glucose through the digestive process. (A smaller amount also comes from protein and fat digestion, but these foods go through their own slower metabolic cycles and do not contribute as much directly to the production of glucose.) Once in the bloodstream, glucose is either used directly to provide energy for our life processes and activities, or it is stored in several ways. It may be stored as glycogen in the liver or in the muscles, or it may be converted to fat and stored as adipose tissue.

The level of glucose in the circulating blood is maintained very precisely in nondiabetics by the interaction of a number of hormones. They increase or decrease the blood sugar level to keep it between 60 and 120 mg/dl. These hormones act in response to a variety of factors, primarily food or lack of food, exercise, and stress (including illness and emotional stress). When the pancreas senses an increase in blood sugar, it releases insulin, which in turn enables glucose molecules to enter cells that would remain closed without it—closed and without fuel.

This spontaneous release of insulin is what we lose when we develop type I diabetes. Blood sugar goes to very high levels (sometimes up to ten times the normal level) because the pancreas releases too little insulin or no insulin. Without adequate insulin, the glucose molecules are unable to pass through the cell walls, and the cells start burning fats instead. This is not as efficient a process as sugar metabolism, and the by-products—ketones—contribute to the ill feelings usually present when diabetes is first diagnosed. Once discovered, type I diabetes must be treated with injected insulin to supplement or replace the insulin from the pancreas.

But insulin is only one of the hormones affecting blood sugar level. Several others work to raise and lower the amount of circulating glucose. Glucagon, also produced by the pancreas, stimulates the release of glucose from the liver. (This substance is available for treatment of reactions when a person is unconscious.) Low blood sugar or stress hormones cue the pancreas to discharge glucagon into the bloodstream. The hormones released when we are under stress include cortisol and epinephrine, both from the adrenal gland. In addition to stimulating glucagon, they have a direct effect on inhibiting the action of insulin. A fourth major factor that also opposes the action of insulin is growth hormone, released by the pituitary gland.

In a nondiabetic, these various hormones work together, raising and lowering blood sugar from moment to moment, so that the proper level is maintained. When activity increases, they increase the glucose available to support it. When a person is under stress, they ensure that the muscles and nervous systems are supplied with enough glucose to function at peak. After eating, the balance shifts so the influx of glucose will be assimilated.

When diabetes develops, insulin, the hormone most important in lowering blood sugar, is no longer available in adequate supply. The others continue to flow freely, however, and contribute to the dramatic increase in blood sugar level. Even when insulin therapy is begun, there isn't the same spontaneous interaction between insulin and other glucose-increasing hormones. The insulin is usually given in fixed amounts rather than in the minutely measured doses the body delivers in response to moment-to-moment need. The automatic feedback loop between blood sugar level and insulin release is broken. The only thing that can begin to replace it is a conscious feedback process requiring external testing of blood (or, a poor second, urine), and decisions about insulin dosage, food, and activity based on test results.

Research scientists and medical engineers are attempting to create devices that will artificially restore the automatic loop. Though good progress is being made, these devices are probably years from general availability. For now, we have the challenge of playing an active and conscious role in one of nature's more elegant processes. We could do worse.

3d. Understand the Factors Determining Blood Sugar Level

Metabolism is an internal process that is continually responding to external factors. Diet, activity level, insulin, dosage, emotional stress, and physical stress all have a powerful influence on our sugar metabolism and the resulting blood sugar levels. Before we can effectively control these levels, we must know why they go up and down as they do. We will review each of the factors influencing blood sugar level and then explore how they work together. (Here we discuss only their effect on blood sugar. Later we discuss other ways they are important in diabetes management.)

Knowledge of how these factors influence blood sugar level allows us to analyze a given test result and understand why it was unexpectedly high or low. In the following discussion, we describe the common, day-to-day aspects of each factor; then we consider the aspects that come into play only occasionally or that affect only some of us.

Major Influences on Blood Sugar Level
In Insulin-Dependent Diabetes

Universal (These factors affect all diabetics.)	*Particular (These factors are temporary or affect only certain people.)*
Insulin	
Types	Immunity to insulin action
Dosage	Interaction with other drugs (medicine, alcohol, marijuana, etc.)
Site of injection	
Schedule	High blood sugar levels inhibit action of insulin
Rebound from reactions	
	Too high dosage
Diet	
Total calories	High fat consumption inhibits insulin action
Distribution of calories among fat, carbohydrate, and protein	
Rate of absorption (glycemic index)	
Fiber	
Activity	
Typical level	Exercise increases blood sugar when it is higher than 250 mg/dl
Frequency and level of exercise	
(There is a delayed lowering of blood sugar as well as the immediate effect with strenuous exercise.)	

Stress	
Physical tension/relaxation	Infection, illness, fever and other physical stresses raise blood sugar
Possible increase or decrease caused by emotional stress	
	Growth spurts
	Over- and undereating when stressed

Other	
Overall degree of regularity	Effects of marijuana, cigarettes, alcohol and other reactional drugs
Menstruation, menopause and pregnancy all affect control	
Socioeconomic—Not having enough money for insulin, testing supplies, and proper diet	

Insulin

The effect of injected insulin on blood sugar level depends upon the type(s) of insulin used, the level and schedule of dosage, the site of injection, the timing of injection in relation to meals, the level of blood sugar, and a number of other factors. Variation of any of these factors can be responsible for the changes in blood sugar level you observe.

The *type(s) of insulin* you take determines the pattern of insulin activity in your body throughout the day. A rapid-acting insulin, such as regular, can begin acting as soon as thirty minutes after injection and reaches its peak of action in two to four hours. Its effect is over in six to eight hours. NPH, on the other hand, starts acting in one to four hours, peaks in six to twelve hours, and may be exhausted after twelve to fourteen hours. Each type of insulin has its characteristic profile of action. Often a rapid-acting insulin is combined with an intermediate or long-acting insulin to create a series of insulin peaks matched to mealtimes.

(Human insulin, now available because of genetic engineering, appears to act sooner, peak earlier, and have a shorter duration of action than animal insulin. This is particularly true for the duration of action of human ultralente.)

In addition, each person has an individual pattern of response to insulin. This is why the times in the following table have so great a range. One may find regular insulin taking effect in thirty minutes; another person may wait an hour. The onset of action, peak of action, and duration all vary from one person to another.

You should know the daily pattern of insulin action your present regimen provides. When does each insulin peak for you? How long is it active? Do your mealtimes coincide with the times of maximum insulin activity? (Your physician can help you understand your insulin profile.) Blood sugar testing allows you to adjust insulin dosage and scheduling to obtain excellent matching between your hour-to-hour need for insulin and its availability. In most cases, this requires at least two shots a day.

Timing of Insulin Action (in hours)

Type	Regular	Semilente	NPH	Lente	Ultralente	Protamine
Onset	1/2-1	1-3	1-4	1-4	4-8	4-8
Peak	2-4	2-8	6-12	6-12	16-24	14-24
Duration	4-8	8-16	12-24	18-28	24-36	24-36

Note: Table derived from several sources, each of which gives different figures. Insulin activity varies greatly from person to person and between animal insulin and human insulin, so these times should be used only as guidelines.

The effectiveness of insulin to lower blood sugar is dramatically decreased by *high blood sugar levels*. At normal levels (70-140 mg/dl), one unit of insulin will usually lower blood glucose around 30 mg/dl. With a high level (such as 300 mg/dl), it might take three units of insulin to lower it by the same amount. This is one of the reasons blood sugar levels sometimes skyrocket and remain high for several days. If stress or a food binge pushes tests to high levels and the usual insulin dose is still taken, its effect is inhibited by the excess sugar. Extra insulin at times like this enables you to regain balance.

High fat levels in the blood also reduce the power of insulin to lower blood sugar. In the short run, you may experience a high test after a meal unusually rich in fats but not necessarily high in carbohydrates. The insulin is just not able to do the same amount of work in the presence of excess fat. If your diet is usually high in fat, you might want to consider lowering the fat to increase the effectiveness of your insulin as well as to improve your general cardiovascular health.

A frustrating fact of insulin therapy is the high blood sugar level that often results from having low blood sugar. This is the rebound from an *insulin reaction.* One of the body's responses to the stress of a reaction is to pump out glucagon, which releases glucose from storage in the liver. We may find high blood sugar levels within an hour of hypoglycemia. This can happen even if we don't overeat when treating the reaction. (This spontaneous rebound can be a lifesaver if one passes out from very low blood sugar.) Hypoglycemia caught in an early stage usually doesn't produce this increase.

Occasionally, the rebound effect becomes a regular part of a diabetic regimen. This can occur when an excessive daily dose of insulin results in regular periods of low blood sugar that are not sensed as reactions (usually occurring during sleep). The body's natural defenses bring blood sugar to a point above normal by the morning test, and insulin may be mistakenly increased. (This Somogyi reaction is discussed in Chapter 8.) High levels before breakfast may also be due to a normal physiologic predawn rise in blood sugar (recently called the "dawn phenomenon"). If this is the case, before-dinner or before-bed insulin should be increased. Near-normal 3:00 A.M. blood sugars paired with high before-breakfast sugars suggest the dawn phenomenon. Near-normal bedtime and low-normal or hypoglycemic 3:00 A.M. levels with high prebreakfast levels suggest the Somogyi reaction. If all three levels are high, more insulin in general is probably needed.

Two other variables of insulin usage have a subtler effect: the part of your body where you inject and the timing of the injection relative to when you eat. Being aware of these increases your ability to fine-tune control after you have mastered the basics, but they are not nearly as important as the facts described above, especially in the beginning of your effort to improve control.

The *site of insulin injection* affects the timing of its action. Insulin injected into the abdomen is absorbed most rapidly, in the thigh, most slowly, and in the arm, at a moderate rate. In one experiment, the time of absorption was approximately 60 minutes for the abdomen, 75 minutes for the arm, and 90 minutes for the thigh. These different absorption times can be used practically: Injection in the abdomen when blood sugar is on the high side or when you want to eat soon; in the leg when a meal may be delayed or when blood sugar is quite low. (The usual rotation of injection site is also necessary. Within any area of the body, change the location you give your shot each day.)

If the site of injection is exercised vigorously, absorption is hastened. An arm swinging a tennis racquet or legs pumping while running will quickly activate insulin injected into them. If you are about to exercise and have recently taken an injection, you should be sure to eat before such activity unless blood sugar is high. If you wish to bring down high blood sugar, giving your shot in the part that is exercised will hasten the process.

The *timing of injection* in relation to mealtime is another subtle variable of insulin therapy. Unless blood sugar is below 80 mg/dl, insulin should usually be taken one-half hour to an hour before meals. This allows the insulin to start working about the time your blood glucose starts to increase from the meal. If you wait until just before the meal or after it, blood sugar is already high by the time the insulin starts to take effect. Shorten the wait if you have reactions before or during the meal.

Both *recreational and medical drugs* can have a significant effect on blood sugar level, either increasing or decreasing the effectiveness of insulin or the other hormones that regulate metabolism. Alcoholic beverages, especially when taken on an empty stomach, increase the ability of insulin to lower blood sugar. Alcohol also interferes with the liver's production of glucose. So drinking before a meal, especially if insulin has just been taken, can lead to reactions. After a drink or two, it may become difficult to notice the symptoms of a reaction. Drinking enough to become fully drunk increases risks further. The reduced awareness, nausea, vomiting, and dehydration play havoc with diabetic control and can lead to ketoacidosis or severe reactions.

Clearly, *alcohol* is to be used by a diabetic in moderation and with awareness. Avoid drinking on an empty stomach, or when blood sugar is relatively low, or after strenuous exercise. Accompany a predinner drink with some carbohydrate snacks. Know the carbohydrate content of your favorite beverages and take it into account in your diet. In some cases, alcohol must be avoided completely. This is an important issue to discuss with your doctor.

Marijuana may have a direct effect on blood sugar by breaking down glycogen, a form in which the body stores sugar. Its release increases blood glucose level. There is no doubt about marijuana's other effect: inducing the "munchies." This drug-induced hunger combines with a weakening of inhibitions to wreak havoc with a pot smoker's diet. As with alcohol, pot increases the risk of not noticing the symptoms of an insulin reaction until it is far advanced, because the sensations of the high mask them. The more powerful forms of marijuana carry the added risk of dependency.

Prescription Drug Interactions with Insulin

Many common prescription drugs can have a serious effect on blood sugar level by their interaction with insulin. Some reduce its power to lower blood sugar or otherwise increase blood glucose. These include diuretics such as Lasix or Thiazide, often used to rid the body of excess water for weight reduction. (They should be used in diabetes for heart disease or high blood pressure only.) Isoniazid (an antituberculosis drug) and estrogens or steroids that increase glucose production in the liver are others.

Other drugs add to the hypoglycemic (blood sugar-lowering) effect of insulin, sometimes causing serious insulin reactions. These include anticoagulants (Coumadin); sulfa (Gantrisin); tranquilizers (Thorazine); MAO inhibitors (Nardil and Parnate); and propranolol (Inderal). Propranolol and other "beta blockers" are potentially very dangerous because they minimize the usual signs of an insulin reaction—

sweating and rapid heartbeat. They are used primarily to treat high blood pressure.

The over-the-counter drugs most likely to influence blood sugar are decongestants and antihistamines.

You should ask whether any drugs prescribed for you affect insulin or blood sugar, especially when you go to a doctor other than the one who sees you for your diabetes. Use your blood test results to determine whether you should change your insulin dosage while you are on the medication prescribed.

One last special condition of insulin therapy: some diabetics develop *resistance to injected insulin,* resulting in decreased effectiveness. (In extreme—but rare—cases, insulin dosage has been increased to hundreds of units per day.) Resistance is caused by antibodies the immune system creates in response to impurities in insulin or to the insulin from a particular animal. Today, all insulin is extremely pure. However, anyone who has been taking insulin for several years may have developed some degree of insulin resistance. It can usually be overcome by using human insulin, highly purified insulin, the insulin from a different animal, or any combination of these types. When the change to more highly purified insulin is made, insulin requirements may decrease by as much as one-third.

Summary

The types of insulin, dosage, schedule of injection, and blood glucose level itself are the most important factors influencing blood glucose level. With the intensive regimen, the central goal is having peaks of insulin activity coincide with the times immediately following meals. This is achieved by taking two or more injections of insulin daily, usually mixing rapid-acting and intermediate or long-acting insulins. Each person should be familiar with the pattern of insulin activity provided by his or her regimen.

The action of insulin is inhibited by high blood sugar levels (over 240 mg/dl) or by high fat consumption. When blood sugar is very high, each unit of insulin is less effective.

Because of the delay before insulin starts acting, injections should usually be taken 30 to 60 minutes before meals. The site of injection has a significant effect on the timing of insulin activity, with the abdomen providing the most rapid start, the arm moderate, and the thigh the slowest.

When insulin reactions occur, the low blood sugar level frequently triggers a stress response resulting in high blood sugar, even though one has eaten moderately to treat the reaction.

Insulin's ability to lower blood sugar may be inhibited or increased by interaction with both recreational and prescription drugs. This can result in unexpected high blood sugar tests or reactions.

Diet

The composition and balance of diet is the second major factor affecting blood glucose level.

We can easily see the impact of the total calories consumed on a given day and how they are distributed between meals and snacks. A too-small lunch on the run or a missed snack may bring low blood sugar and a reaction a little later. Overindulgence at one meal results in high tests afterwards. Heavy eating throughout a day may drive blood sugar up for several days if adjustments are not made.

When you are first learning to manage diabetes, a relatively regular pattern of eating, with approximately the same number of calories consumed at the same time each day, is one of the fundamental ingredients. With regular home blood glucose testing, you can determine the results of departures from the norm, and you can learn to correct them by adjusting day-to-day insulin dose and exercise. (Once you have mastered your regimen, it is possible to vary food intake and timing and still maintain good control.)

Another aspect of diet affecting control is the speed at which different foods are converted into blood sugar. Although its utility is still being debated, nutrition researchers have developed a *glycemic index* to measure the conversion rate for different foods. They have found, for instance, that potatoes eaten alone bring a rise in blood sugar as fast as does a drink of glucose syrup. Pasta and beans, on the other hand, are absorbed much more slowly and result in a smaller increase in blood sugar at any one time.

The main categories of food—carbohydrate, fat, and protein—show different absorption times. Simple carbohydrates (sugars and highly refined starches) usually reach the blood stream quickly, peaking in 15 to 30 minutes. Complex carbohydrates (most starchy vegetables, whole grains, and beans) take from 30 to 90 minutes to reach their maximum impact on blood sugar. Fats take around 90 minutes, and proteins, 3 hours. (These times, however, vary greatly among specific foods. Chapter 9 presents a more detailed discussion of this subject.)

A well-balanced meal provides a gradual, sustained input of nutrition, avoiding the sudden high peak of blood sugar that a meal of simple carbohydrates causes. The amount of fiber in our food also affects absorption rate. High-fiber diets tend to slow the rate. High fat content, as indicated above, tends to interfere with the action of insulin, causing a need for higher doses. On the other hand, fat tends to slow the absorption of other foods eaten at the same time.

Significant daily variations in any of these factors—overall calories or balance between different food categories—can result in unexpectedly high or low blood glucose readings. For instance, high blood sugar caused by eating mostly simple carbohydrates may be followed in a short time by a serious reaction. Not enough slowly absorbed food is in the intestine to provide continued, gradual input of blood sugar. Or an overdose of steak and potatoes with butter and sour cream may bring elevated blood sugar the next morning and midday because the food is digested slowly and the fat decreases insulin effectiveness. Knowing how these principles apply to you, supplemented by results of your self blood glucose testing, will help you adjust your control.

Summary

The total calories consumed, how the calories are distributed between meals and snacks, and the types and combinations of foods consumed determine the impact on blood sugar level. Until you have learned the whole management regimen, you should eat approximately the same amounts of food (in terms of calories or exchanges) at approximately the same times each day.

Simple carbohydrates (sugars, fruits, juices, milk) are converted to blood glucose within a few minutes; complex carbohydrates (starchy vegetables, whole grains, and beans) take from thirty to ninety minutes; fats, around ninety minutes and proteins, up to three hours. High-fiber foods are absorbed more slowly and tend to slow the absorption rate of other foods as well. Regular high fat consumption inhibits the action of insulin

A diet high in fiber and relatively low in fat that minimizes consumption of simple carbohydrates results in more stable blood sugar levels, with less severe peaks after meals. This is probably the best disbetes diet.

Activity

This is the third major influence on blood sugar. Control is profoundly affected by the general pattern of movement and exertion we follow as well as any periods of special exercise or work. Changes in either type or activity usually bring increases or decreases in blood sugar level and may result in insulin reactions. As with the other major factors determining blood level, the more regular you are in your daily activities, the easier it will be for you to achieve optimal control.

General physical activity and specific times of exercise affect blood sugar in several ways. There is the immediate lowering due to the energy spent. The more strenuous the exercise, the faster blood glucose goes down. If insulin has not been decreased or food increased, a reaction is likely to occur (unless blood sugar level is high to begin with). Furthermore, during and following exercise, additional decreases in blood sugar level occur as the muscles absorb and store glucose beyond what they are burning. This process may continue for several hours after you have exercised vigorously. For this reason, reactions may occur long after you have finished the activity. Glucose is being pulled out of the bloodstream by muscles that need to replenish their stores.

Once you have learned to adjust diet and insulin dose, it becomes easier to avoid heavy reactions caused by exercise. In fact, the increased glucose storage means you will enjoy more stability of your blood sugar level. When it starts to fall, more glucose is available to bring it back up to normal spontaneously.

If you maintain an active life, especially if you are able to follow a consistent, conditioning program, there is an added benefit: your sensitivity to insulin is increased. This means that a given amount of exercise will lower your blood sugar more and a unit of insulin will be more effective. Insulin dose can be cut by a few units, more if you were sedentary before. A conditioning program is an exercise regimen in which you reach your peak of physical functioning three times a week for a least twenty minutes. Breathing is full and pulse is at the level defined for your age.

You don't have to exercise strenuously to gain benefits from physical activity. Even moderate movement—a quiet walk or work in the garden—can have a significant effect on blood sugar levels, compared to sitting and reading or watching television. This is important, as you may need to avoid heavy exercise. If complications have developed, you may experience severe harm from exercise programs that fail to respect your physical limitations. Especially if you have early signs of complications, you should discuss your exercise program with your doctor.

Ironically, the power of exercise to reduce blood sugar is destroyed when the level is higher than 250 or 300 mg/dl, especially if ketones are present. When we need it most, the effect of exercise is reversed and blood sugar increases. *If your blood sugar level is higher than 250 mg/dl, especially when acetone tests are positive, do not try to bring it down with exercise.* At this level your body doesn't perform well and you won't enjoy it, anyway.

Summary

Physical activity helps to lower and stabilize blood sugar levels, with the greatest benefits gained from regular exercise. Changes in activity level must be balanced by corresponding adjustments of diet or insulin dose in order to avoid serious reactions. When complications are developing, medical guidance in choosing appropriate physical activity is absolutely necessary.

Chapter 10, "Living Actively With Diabetes," gives more detail on all of these subjects.

Stress

Stress is the fourth major influence on blood sugar level. When we are presented with any challenge, physical or emotional, we adapt to it through a complex set of chemical and muscular changes. This physical adaptation is what we call the stress response, something neither negative nor positive in itself. (The noted student of stress, Hans Selye, draws a distinction between *distress*, "negative" stress, and *eustress*, "good" stress.) We need the stress response to function; it mobilizes us for action and organizes our defenses to maintain vital functions when we are ill or injured. However, in diabetes one aspect of the stress response itself becomes a challenge. To protect the brain and ensure energy for action, stress produces a rapid change of blood sugar level, often an increase.

Perhaps you have experienced a severe flu in which your urine or blood sugar tests were high even though you ate little. This is a classic example of the diabetic stress response triggered by a physical disorder. Other *physical stressors* include injury, burns, infections, severe pain, dehydration, surgery, hypothermia (extreme chill), exhausting exercise, and insulin reactions. These triggers cause blood sugar to soar, insulin to be less effective, and if the condition persists, toxic ketones to build up in the bloodstream.

If you experience any of these physical stresses, you should carefully monitor your response by frequently testing your blood sugar and urine ketones, continue taking insulin, with extra injections of regular as needed, and contact your physician if you do not return to normal blood sugar levels and absence of ketones within a day. You may be in danger of going into ketoacidosis (diabetic coma) if any serious physical disorder is not handled properly. The risk is small if you act immediately to compensate for the effect of these disorders on your control.

You don't have to feel seriously ill for a physical stress to have a strong effect on your blood sugar level; so when you have a high test that you can't explain, check to see if anything is happening with your body that might be causing the increase—an infected cut, a bad sunburn, or fatigue, for example.

Emotions, images, and ideas can trigger the stress response as surely as a physical disorder. In fact, the body can't really tell the difference. An argument, a disappointment, even a thrilling discovery may bring about release of hormones that raise or lower blood sugar, sometimes dramatically. A sense of frustration or depression that continues for days may mean elevated blood sugar throughout the period. (The effect we are describing here is independent of any nervous nibbling of extra food you may indulge in during stressful times. This habit adds to the hormonal effects of stress to produce even higher blood sugar levels.)

So stress is one more variable to help you understand why your test results change when you think you are following your regimen carefully. With an awareness of the role of stress in your life, you are equipped to adjust for its effects on your metabolism (and even control it).

Unfortunately, there have been few clear research findings on the way emotional stress affects diabetic management. Like many other aspects of our condition, stress appears to be highly individual in its effects. Some people show relatively little change in blood sugar level after stressful experiences. Others experience amazing increases in blood sugar, and some find that it drops when they are under stress. The effect may depend on the type of emotion aroused, the duration and intensity of the experience, one's ability to express the feelings through communication or action, and the level of blood sugar at the time the incident begins.

You can use your blood glucose testing to do your own research on emotional stress in diabetes. When you have had a difficult day at work or school, an argument, a fright, or a strong disappointment, check your blood sugar level. See if it is significantly higher or lower than what you would expect on the basis of the day's activity and food. Some find that a stressful experience can raise blood sugar to the 400s, even higher. Note, too, whether you tend to have reactions after particular kinds of stress, especially those in which you have expressed your feelings strongly. A decrease in blood sugar level is also possible. Keeping notes on your observations in a section of your diabetes log is helpful. After a while, you will have a clearer picture of how your system responds to emotional stress.

Diabetics who experience chronically high stress levels in daily life often find that their blood sugar level decreases when they give themselves permission to relax. A holiday or vacation may bring more insulin reactions, not only because of increased exercise, but also because greater calmness means that fewer stress hormones (which counteract insulin) are at work. Studies are beginning to demonstrate that regular periods of relaxation can lower insulin requirements for many diabetics.

Summary

Severe physical stress, occurring as the result of illness, infection, or injury, increases blood sugar levels and the development of ketones in the blood and urine. Careful monitoring of blood sugar and urine ketone levels and consultation with a physician are recommended when a person with diabetes encounters such stress.

Emotional stress may raise or lower blood sugar levels, depending on a number of factors. (It can also stimulate the development of ketones.) Each diabetic needs to observe his or her own pattern of response to stress and learn to adjust insulin, food, and exercise accordingly. Stress management and relaxation training can reduce the impact of stress on diabetic control.

Hormonal Changes in Women

Menstruation, pregnancy, and menopause trigger change in hormone levels that in turn affect control for diabetic women (see Chapter 18). Variations in control during a woman's menstrual period have only recently been noted in diabetes care books. Unfortunately, little systematic research has been done. It appears from personal reports that the impact on blood sugar levels varies from woman to woman and at different phases of a woman's period. So this is another place in which the woman with diabetes becomes her own researcher. Use your blood sugar tests to see whether there are changes just before and during your menstrual period. You may need to make modest changes in insulin or food intake to compensate.

The many physical changes occurring in the pregnant woman with diabetes include an initial reduction in insulin requirement, and, after the first two or three months, an increase. Every stage of pregnancy should be supervised by a physician who has worked with diabetic pregnancies and is thoroughly committed to maintaining optimal control.

During menopause, profound hormonal changes occur that can affect blood sugar levels. Unfortunately, little research information is available, and the influences seem to vary from woman to woman. There is also the hazard of mistaking hot flashes for insulin reactions, and vice versa. This is a time when home blood testing can help a woman avoid confusion.

Puberty

During puberty, many physical and emotional changes affect blood sugar levels profoundly. In some cases, insulin dosage may have to be doubled to compensate for the impact of shifts in hormone levels. When teen rebellion is added to the mix, going through puberty calls for special strategies for teens with diabetes and their families.

Summary of Step 3d

All these factors work together. The interaction among them is, of course, what finally determines your blood sugar level at any time. Sometimes different factors balance each other, and sometimes they add to each other's effect, causing a steep rise or fall.

After a period of intense jogging, you may still find a high blood sugar level if you were extremely stressed because someone almost ran over you. On the other hand, if you ate only quickly absorbed carbohydrates before jogging, you may have a severe reaction an hour or two later because the blood sugar was burnt up during exercise and no reserves remain.

If you get depressed because blood sugar tests have been high, the emotional reaction may drive them still higher. If you don't adjust insulin dosage to deal with the high level, each unit is less effective and blood sugar may go up even more.

This all sounds very complex. However, if you are willing to stabilize as many factors as possible during this period of learning the intensive regimen, you will soon be able to sort out which influences on blood sugar are at work at any given time. This is the reason for the next task.

Step 4: Regularize diet, activity, and schedules during the learning period

This temporary step of regularizing your life allows much more freedom in diabetes management in the long run. While learning the intensive regimen, you should eat more or less the same number of calories (or food exchanges) in each meal and snack; maintain a similar activity and exercise level from day to day; keep insulin dosage the same until instructed to alter it according to your tests; and not vary the timing of injections or meals by more than an hour.

Without this step, you will find it very difficult to understand how your system responds to the many variables affecting metabolic control. If diet, activity, schedules, and stress are all changing each day, you will lack the stability needed to establish the best insulin dosage or to learn how to vary insulin, diet, and activity to compensate for blood sugar levels that are too high or too low.

After a few months of following this routine carefully, it is possible to live with much less regularity and still keep blood sugar tests within limits. You will have learned how your system functions, how the different ingredients of your regimen affect you, and how to vary them to obtain good control.

You may also have learned some internal cues that alert you to your level of control. You will understand what has caused a particular high test or insulin reaction; and you will have greater ability to make changes each day to even out the highs and lows. A relatively brief period of increased regularity will give you a life of greater freedom.

This step does not mean you should become rigid or compulsive and create a new source of stress in your life. Keep things as regular as you can from day to day, and see the times when diet or activity does change a lot as opportunities to study the effects of the changes on your blood sugar. (Remember, this is guilt-free learning.) Give yourself permission to take a day or two off from the routine now and then. You will return to it with renewed discipline. The changes you are making will last if you achieve them through willingness rather than force.

Some people may find it difficult to achieve greater regularity, either because of outside demands or because of their own emotional reactions. Work schedules and levels of activity may change frequently; regular daily exercise may not fit into already busy lives; or one may simply want to retain previous ideas of what freedom is.

If you do not find it easy to make your life more systematic, even for a few months, you can still improve control to an extent. Test as often as possible and record your results, together with notes on diet, activity, and stress. By reviewing the patterns in your records with your doctor or diabetes educator, you will get a better idea of what makes blood sugar rise and fall in your case. You are also likely to become more willing to become more regular: You will have precise evidence of the effects of your lack of routine. (If you would like to explore the reasons for your reluctance, use the exercises in Chapters 3 and 14.)

One way of making this period of increased regularity more acceptable is to offer yourself a reward. For some people, the benefits of improved control are reward enough. But you may find it easier to reinforce your motivation by agreeing to give yourself some special experience or gift. After so many weeks of straight-arrow living, you become eligible for that trip or event or object you have been wishing for. Children like rewards, and we need to cooperate with the child within us to maintain discipline (see Chapter 2).

Step 5: Begin period of intensive testing and record keeping

Many of us experience a sense of excitement as we begin testing blood sugar at home. For the first time, we are able to observe exactly how our system is affected by the food we eat, exercise (or inactivity), and the stresses we experience. We can find out if that queasy feeling is an insulin reaction or a stress response (or just an unexplained queasy feeling). We can measure the effect of "just a few cookies" or extra slices of fresh bread and butter. We have the feedback essential to living well with diabetic control.

At the start, your doctor will probably ask you just to observe the pattern of blood sugar readings without making any changes in regimen. You will need to record tests for several days, along with detailed notes on food, exercise, stress, and any changes that might affect your tests. (Use one of the logs in Step 3.) In this first period, your learning will be most rapid if you test before every insulin injection, before each meal, one to two hours after each meal, and at bedtime. In addition, test your blood sugar when you suspect that you are having an insulin reaction. If you show any signs of having reactions while sleeping, set the alarm and test around 2:00 or 3:00 in the morning (see Chapter 8 for signs of Somogyi reactions).

This may sound like a lot of finger pricks (up to seven or eight a day), but testing this often is necessary for only a few weeks, and the information you gain is pure gold. With it you and your physician will be able to tailor your insulin, diet, and activity to achieve great improvements in your level of metabolic control.

It is useful to assume the role of a scientific observer, not a judge of right and wrong, as you observe your test results. You are likely to find the jumps in blood sugar level puzzling at first. Many of us fall into the trap of believing that "I must have done something wrong." You will learn faster if you simply record the results (even if it is the result of a binge) and go on from there, without blame. Record all of your tests and don't neglect tests because you already know they will be high. It will help you to see how high they actually are. You are in the process of learning to control blood sugar. You can't possibly have it all under control yesterday.

Step 6: Selecting the ongoing insulin regimen
With your initial blood tests in hand, you and your doctor are now ready to decide what (if any) changes are needed in your insulin regimen—the types, dosage, and timing of insulin you take. The

insulin regimen chosen must be capable of meeting the following criteria.

Criteria for Insulin Regimen

1. Timing and dosage of insulin delivery provides for continuous, low-level availability of insulin throughout the twenty-four hours as well as peaks of insulin action following meals.

2. The majority of tests are between 70 and 150 mg/dl.

3. Hemoglobin A_1c is below 9.

4. Insulin reactions are not frequent, and their impact is minimized.

5. Normal body weight is maintained (excess weight is lost).

6. Flexibility in dealing with day-to-day changes and stress is ensured.

7. The convenience and preference of the individual diabetic are respected.

8. In children, normal growth and development are maintained.

A variety of insulin regimens are available that satisfy these criteria: two, three or four injections a day, with or without mixtures of different types of insulin, or the continuous infusion of insulin provided by the pump. With these alternatives, it is possible to tailor the pattern of insulin action more precisely to meet your individual needs.

Determining the Total Insulin Dose

Recommended starting levels for intensive insulin regimens are as follows:

1. In newly diagnosed patients: 0.5 units of insulin per kilogram per day (132-pound person weighs 60 kg; 0.5 x 60 = 30 units of insulin per day).

2. During the "honeymoon" period, when insulin requirements temporarily decrease for the new diabetic: 0.4 units per kg per day.

3. For established patients previously treated with more than 0.9 units per kilogram per day: reduce dose by 20 to 25 percent. (A 132-pound person taking 60 units would reduce dose by 12 to 15 units.)

4. For patients previously treated with 0.7 to 0.9 units per kilogram per day: use 0.7 units per kilogram per day.

5. For patients previously treated with less than 0.7 units per kilogram per day: use old total dose unless it obviously is inadequate.

These are general guidelines, developed from averages for many patients. Your specific dosage will be worked out with your physician, taking your unique needs into account. We are providing the information so you will know what is happening, not because this is a do-it-yourself step.

Your total daily insulin dosage is the first thing to be determined with your physician. When changing from a single daily injection to a more intensive treatment plan, insulin requirements change, usually downward. The total dosage of insulin you take each day is determined by your body weight and general level of activity.

For diabetics within 20 percent of ideal body weight and without illness or high levels of emotional stress, the daily dose varies between 0.5 and 1.0 unit of insulin for each kilogram of weight (1 kilogram = 2.2 pounds; 150 lb. divided by 2.2 = 70 kg).

After the daily dosage of insulin is determined, your physician will recommend one or two types of insulin, distributed into two or more injections a day. Many studies have been completed attempting to find the best style of treatment. So far it appears that the specific insulin regimen is not nearly as important as the total program of self-care. One research project in Florida compared the control of patients using the insulin pump, twice-a-day injections, and four-times-a-day injections. Their home and lab tests indicated excellent control on all three regimens. The researchers concluded that selection of insulin regimen could be a matter of patient preference. Patient success was based on the full intensive regimen, not just the insulin regimen.

So it appears that you are free to choose the intensive insulin regimen that fits with your personal style if you are willing to follow all the other parts of the full intensive regimen. (In some cases, special factors may make one regimen more effective than another. Your physician will discuss these with you if any apply to you.) The critical elements are your awareness and willingness to make adjustments each day to maintain optimal control.

Insulin Regimens For Optimal Control

1. Two injections of intermediate (NPH or Lente) and rapid-acting insulin taken before breakfast and before dinner.

2. Three injections: intermediate and rapid in morning, rapid before dinner, intermediate at bedtime.

3. Three injections: rapid and Ultralente before breakfast and dinner, rapid before lunch.

4. Four injections: rapid before meals and intermediate at bedtime.

5. The insulin pump provides both a continuous low-level flow of insulin and boluses or bursts of insulin before meals.

These regimens have been used and studied in research trials. Other dosage programs can be developed that may better suit your individual needs. The variety of insulins now available allows you to work with your doctor to find a mix that functions best for you.

(The convenience of the single-injection regimen is its only advantage, so it will be discussed later, in the sections on moderate and loose regimens. For anyone seeking optimal control, at least two shots a day with a mix of intermediate and rapid-acting insulins are required.)

Some people dislike injections and resist the idea of taking several a day. An alternative of injections with a syringe and needle is the jet, or needleless, injection, using an instrument that injects insulin at high pressure through the skin's surface.

Gary Does Away with the Needle

I have been using a jet injector (Medijector) for over fifteen years. I began using it initially because of curiosity and the hope that it would make my life somewhat easier. (I didn't particularly dislike injections after twenty years of them). I found this method of taking insulin faster and more convenient.

For people interested in avoiding the pain of the needle, jet injection is generally more comfortable. For me, the occasional discomfort is associated with larger volume of insulin, type of insulin, or tougher skin.

Another benefit of the jet injector is reduction in insulin dose due to improved absorption. When I switched to it, I could cut my dose in half. Most people don't experience such dramatic changes.

If you are thinking of switching to jet injection, you should consult your physician, because it requires a prescription. The relatively high price is covered by most medical insurance. But if it isn't, it can pay for itself over time, compared to the cost of disposable needles. (The device I use is the Medi-Jector® made by Derata Corp. in Minneapolis. They are a very reliable and committed company.)

When two or more injections are taken each day, it is possible to adjust the peaks of insulin activity and the ongoing insulin availability to your individual life pattern. In fact, this individualization is essential. Your physician and you will use your home blood sugar tests to determine the best pattern for you. With care you can have near-normal blood sugar levels throughout the day. When tests are high, you can take action to bring blood sugar down.

The Regimens

1. The least demanding insulin regimen is the two-injection plan, in which rapid acting (regular) and intermediate (NPH or Lente) insulins are taken thirty to sixty minutes before breakfast and dinner. (In the Florida study, two-thirds of the total dose was taken before breakfast, with two-thirds of the shot intermediate insulin, and one-third regu-

lar.) The predinner shot was equal parts of the two insulins. Your doctor will select your dose according to your test results, and your meal and activity patterns.) The peaks of the regular insulin handle the increase in blood sugar caused by breakfast and dinner. The peaks of the intermediate insulin cover lunch and the overnight need.

The more gradual action of the intermediate provides continuing low-level insulin activity. The greater convenience is the major advantage of this regimen. Its disadvantage is that one has less flexibility in the timing and size of lunch. If tests are high at midday, an extra shot of regular may be needed.

Two Injections Before Breakfast and Dinner

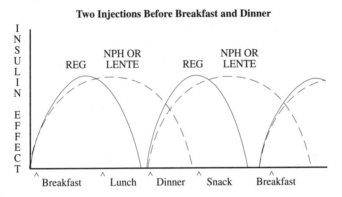

2. The second plan is essentially a variation of the first. The main difference is that the evening shot is divided, with rapid-acting insulin taken before dinner and intermediate at bedtime. This allows better overnight coverage for those who need more low-level insulin action while they sleep in order to wake up with a normal blood sugar level. It has the same disadvantage as plan 1.

Three Injections Intermediate and Rapid

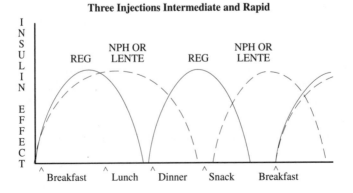

3. Plan 3 requires three injections daily, with a mixture of regular (or Semilente) and Ultralente twenty to thirty minute before breakfast and dinner, and regular only before lunch. (Here the long-acting Ultralente makes up 40 to 50 percent of the total dosage. The regular is divided equally between the three shots.) The regular insulin covers meals and the Ultralente ensures continuing low-level supply of insulin throughout the twenty-four hours.

This regimen provides a great deal of flexibility, allowing one to change mealtime or size and activity plans, and to correct for high blood sugar levels before each meal. (This is helpful for shift workers or people with schedules that change often.) The chief disadvantage lies with the very long time of action of each Ultralente injection. It takes approximately four days to determine the effect of a change in dosage. Furthermore, the rate of absorption of this insulin varies, which can result in periods of sustained hypoglycemia. Probably this regimen is advisable only when your physician has extensive experience with the ins and outs of Ultralente.[1]

Three Injections Rapid and Ultralente

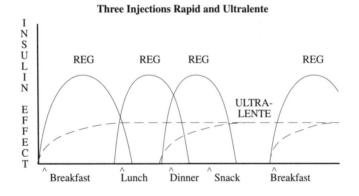

Gary's Ultralente Anecdote

My personal experience using Ultralente is only a case history. There is little direct support for it in the diabetes literature.

[1] From Jay Skyler, "Type I Diabetes...Regimens, Targets, and Caveats: Diabetes Care, 5(5):550 (1982).

Currently I take one injection of animal Ultralente each morning. I supplement the Ultralente with regular insulin only when I am planning to have a large meal or otherwise find my blood sugar too high, and I have reasonably good control over twenty-four-hour periods. I have not been bothered by the reported unpredictable time of action of Ultralente, and I find the extra duration of coverage into the next day very helpful in preventing early-morning hyperglycemia. I like the combination of convenience and control that I can obtain with this regimen. It is certainly not for everybody.

I began using Ultralente insulin many years before it became medically fashionable. I found that I could obtain better control with fewer reactions (either late in the afternoon or early in the morning) using only Ultralente than with mixtures of Lente and Semilente. Since Lente insulin was at the time a fixed-ratio mixture of 30 percent Semilente and 70 percent Ultralente (currently, I believe Lente is formulated directly to produce that combination of activity, rather than as a mixture of the two), I started mixing Semi and Ultra to find the ratio that worked for me. As I adjusted the amounts, I found that I was gradually decreasing the Semi and increasing the Ultra. Finally, all I was taking was Ultralente. Thus, before anyone had written about using Ultra for "basal" insulin levels, I was using it as my only insulin. My own experience, personal and anecdotal, suggests that it is an underused insulin. Increasing attention is being paid to it, particularly the differences in the peaks and duration of action between human and animal Ultralente, and the need for longer action of human Ultralente.[2,3,4]

[2] D.E. Seigler, et al., "Pharmacokinetics of long acting (ultralente) insulin preparations," Diabetes Nutrition and Metabolism, 4(4): 1-7 (1991).

[3] M. Parillo, et al., "Prevention of early morning hyperglycemia in IDDM patients with long-acting zinc insulin," Diabetes Care, 15(2): 173-177 (Feb 1992).

[4] M. Albisser & M. Sperlich, "Adjusting insulins," The Diabetes Educator, 18(3): 211-222 (May/June 1992).

If one of you is interested in trying this, I suggest you discuss it with your physician and work out a program that you monitor carefully. Perhaps you will start with one of the more typical patterns, using Ultralente (once or twice a day with regular before meals, as needed). Home blood glucose testing makes it a lot easier to figure out what is working well for you.

One additional caution: The human Ultralente insulins have a shorter duration of action than the animal insulins. If you are presently taking human insulin and have never taken animal, it's probably best to stick with human and see if the human Ultralente gives you long enough coverage. If you're taking animal insulin now or have taken it in the past, it's probably fine to try the longer-acting animal Ultralente. Discuss this with your doctor. Animal insulins are much purer now than they were several years ago, and the antibodies you may have to animal insulin will probably not be a factor for you.

Ernest Becomes an Ultralente Convert

My earlier regimen of NPH and regular insulin before breakfast and dinner started producing unacceptable results when I increased my daily exercise. Various small adjustments failed to achieve normal blood sugar in the morning. After discussion with Gary and my regular physician, I shifted to an Ultralente and regular mix before breakfast and dinner. The result: fewer reactions and better balance throughout the day.

4. The fourth insulin regimen includes three injections of rapid-acting insulin thirty minutes before meals and one of the intermediate-acting (NPH or Lente) at bedtime. This plan allows one to adjust dose to meal size and every meal, but meals must not be greatly delayed or blood sugar may rise. This is because the regular dosage, which covers each meal, is declining in action by the next meal. The intermediate insulin before bed provides the additional low-level insulin action needed while asleep. The distribution of total insulin dosage throughout the day is highly individualized and is best left to be determined by your physician and your blood glucose patterns.

Four Injections

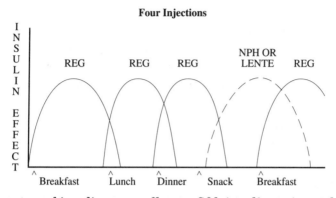

5. The external insulin pump allows a fifth insulin regimen that comes closest to the natural pattern of insulin availability found in the nondiabetic. The device feeds a small amount of insulin at regular intervals into the abdomen through a tube and needle (or catheter) that remain implanted day and night. (The needle must be changed every one to three days. New devices allow the needle to be removed immediately after insertion, leaving behind a soft, flexible tube.) Before a meal or snack, the user triggers a measured burst or "bolus" of extra insulin to handle the increase in blood sugar from the food. The most advanced models contain microcomputer chips that allow setting different rates of delivery for waking and sleeping hours.

Insulin Pump

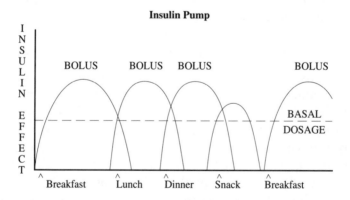

Even though the insulin-pump user may be wearing a tiny computer, this innovation still demands a very active role in management. Four to seven blood tests each day are recommended as standard procedure;

these allow adjustment of the premeal boluses to actual blood sugar level. The person using the pump must also be especially aware of reactions (whose warning signs may become quite subtle) and the danger of fairly sudden rises in blood sugar through malfunction.

Many of us have willingly become pump users, experiencing improved control and a wide range of side effects. Wearing a device that is plugged into one's belly (with some models that beep regularly) is a constant reminder of diabetes. This reminder can become physically painful if infection develops at the hookup site—not an unusual complication. The danger of hypoglycemia is greater because it is so easy to take extra insulin with the pump. This also results in a tendency for pump users to gain weight, especially at the beginning. Being a machine, the pump is subject to malfunction. Its foibles have caused both severe insulin reactions and ketoacidosis.

In spite of the side effects and the cost ($2,000 to $3,000), thousands are now using the insulin pump. Rapid progress is being made on overcoming its relatively infrequent technical failings, and greatly improved models will probably be on the market by the time you read this. It is clearly a viable choice for the person who wishes to maintain optimal control. If you are interested, discuss it with your physician and with people who are actually using a pump. But remember, it is not a replacement for your active participation in the management of your diabetes.

Currently in the research and development phase are implantable (internal) pumps about the size of a hockey puck, which are inserted under the skin. Concentrated insulin is injected monthly through the skin into the pump, and the pump is programmed by a hand-held remote-controlled device.

MAKING THE CHOICE

Now the art of medicine comes into play. There is no formula for prescribing insulin regimen. This is a highly individual process that takes into account the pattern of your test records, your personal style and preferences, your daily schedule, and even the style of your physician. Over the course of several weeks, you and your physician will work together, most likely with a phone consultation every few days, to adjust the initial dosage. Your test results and insulin reactions will provide the feedback needed to fine-tune the regimen and achieve blood sugar levels within the limits the two of you have agreed on. (If you are very loosely controlled to begin with, these may be higher than the optimal level for the first months and gradually brought down.) For many doctors and patients alike, the teamwork that develops at this stage is highly rewarding. If, on the other hand, your doctor gives little guidance at this stage, you may need to search for one who is either more knowledgeable or more cooperative.

The general guidelines for adjusting insulin regimen include the following:

1. Normalize the fasting blood sugar level first by adjusting the overnight insulin. Increase it only after determining that night-time reactions are not the cause of high fasting blood glucose tests. (See "Somogyi Reactions" in Chapter 8.)

2. When changes in dosage are needed, change only one type of insulin given at a particular time of day. (Determine the overall effect of changing morning NPH, for instance, before changing morning regular or dosage at other times.)

3. Wait two to three days to see the effect of the change before making any further change. (Wait three to four days with Ultralente insulin.)

4. Dosage should not be changed more than one unit at a time for anyone under 90 pounds.

5. For those over 90 pounds, increases of insulin should generally be one to two units at a time, although changes of two to six units may be made if your doctor advises.

6. Adjustments in dosage should be made on the basis of a pattern found over several days of testing, not just because of one high test or reaction.

7. Check for Somogyi reaction if results of changes are opposite what you would expect. If insulin is increased (or food decreased) and

blood sugar goes up, high tests may indicate a rebound from too much insulin.

By the time you have established your ongoing insulin regimen, you will have some understanding of the timing of each insulin component—when it peaks and what meal it covers. The timing of reactions will help you sense this timing. You will also begin to know the art of making adjustments in dosage to keep your tests within the target range you are aiming for.

If your activity level changes significantly from weekday to weekend, you may need to adjust your dosage regularly to account for the change. Women may need to make adjustments when menstruation affects blood sugar levels. Workers with swing or graveyard shifts may need regular shifts in insulin. In the beginning, check with your physician before making such changes. As you become experienced, you will probably be encouraged to take the initiative.

If you experience a major improvement in control at this stage, with the majority of your tests in the target range, you may feel uncomfortable for a short time. At first, you may even have symptoms of hypoglycemia when your blood sugar level is normal. This is natural while you adjust to the new level of control. Discomfort can last up to two weeks. When your system gets used to the new level, you will feel better than you ever did when blood sugar was chronically high.

If, on the other hand, you find it difficult to bring your tests within the range you would like or if there is a great fluctuation in readings, don't despair. There can be many reasons for the frustration you experience, and there are just as many solutions. At this point, the next step is discovering the reason and defining what has to be done to correct the problem. Skip to Step 9 at this point to clarify the cause of your difficulty and what you need to do to get past it.

Step 7: Observe the variations in blood sugar level caused by changes in food and exercise, stress, illness, and other factors.

You will, of course, start to observe the causes of blood sugar variations as soon as you begin testing. But now it will be easier to sort out the factor or factors causing a particular high or low reading. In Step 3, you reviewed all of the influences at work here, and this information will be put to work at this point. Your doctor may prefer that you spend some time just observing before you start making changes to compensate for levels outside your target range. Or you may begin making cautious changes right away, in which case you will be doing the two parts of Step 7 at the same time.

Look through the sample logs that follow and see how many of the high tests or reactions you can explain. Then read the discussion of each log.

Daily Diabetes Log

Susan is on insulin regimen 1, with a regular dose of 15 NPH and 4 regular before breakfast, 10 NPH and 5 regular before dinner.

DATE & TIME	BLOOD TEST & REAC- TIONS	INSULIN DOSAGE	ACTIVITY & EXERCISE	FOOD	COMMENTS: Stress, illness, etc.
8-15 7 AM	110	15 NPH 5 reg	walk 30 min	8 AM 2 bread 1 oz cheese orange	
10 AM					My boss blew up at me for losing an important account. I felt guilty & angry and just stewed.
11:45 AM	240 (a)			Green salad & ham	Cut the carbo for lunch.

DATE & TIME	BLOOD TEST & REAC- TIONS	INSULIN DOSAGE	ACTIVITY & EXERCISE	FOOD	COMMENTS: Stress, illness, etc.
4 PM	#2 react (b)			Pack of choco- late cookies	
5:30 PM	200(c)	10 NPH 7 reg	Walk 30 min	One cup rice 3 oz ham- burg yellow squash 3 plums	Quiet evening
10 PM	120			1 bread 1 oz peanut butter	

Before reading on, give your explanation of the high tests at (a) and (c) and the reaction at (b). What, if anything, could Susan have done to avoid them? What did she do to compensate?

Susan's high blood sugar level at lunch was probably caused by the emotional stress of being disciplined by her boss and not feeling able to express her feelings. Probably nothing short of a deep pool of inner peace could have spared her this high test. She then overcompensated for the high reading by avoiding carbohydrates altogether at lunch rather than just reducing them.

Her roller coaster went from high to low, resulting in the reaction at 4:00 P.M. Rebound from the strong reaction (and probably an overdose of chocolate cookies) caused another high blood sugar level at 5:30. One can do nothing to avoid rebound, but not overtreating reactions helps lessen the rise in blood sugar. An additional two units of regular (over her usual five units) and a thirty-minute walk allowed Susan to return to a blood sugar level within her target range by bedtime.

Managing your blood sugar choices

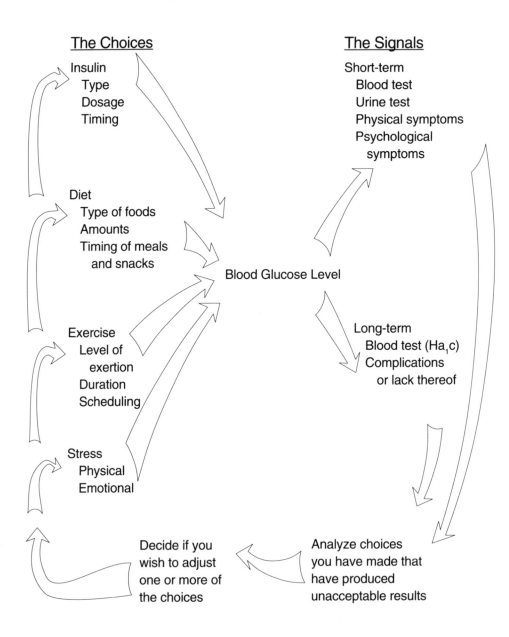

The Choices

Insulin
   Type
   Dosage
   Timing

Diet
   Type of foods
   Amounts
   Timing of meals
    and snacks

Exercise
   Level of
    exertion
   Duration
   Scheduling

Stress
   Physical
   Emotional

The Signals

Short-term
   Blood test
   Urine test
   Physical symptoms
   Psychological
    symptoms

Blood Glucose Level

Long-term
   Blood test (Ha$_1$c)
   Complications
    or lack thereof

Decide if you
wish to adjust
one or more of
the choices

Analyze choices
you have made that
have produced
unacceptable results

Daily Diabetes Log

George is on regimen 3. His standard dosage is 8 units of Ultralente and 7 units of regular before breakfast and dinner, and 7 units of regular before lunch.

DATE & TIME	BLOOD TEST & REAC- TIONS	INSULIN DOSAGE	ACTIVITY & EXERCISE	FOOD	COMMENTS: Stress, illness, etc.
Mar 5 6:30 AM	90	8 ultr 7 reg		7 AM cup Oatmeal Cup milk 1 oz raisins 1 oz cashews	
7:30 AM			Jogging 45 min		
11 AM	mild reac(a)			Orange juice	
12 noon	140(b)	8 reg		Egg salad sandwich Med apple	Headache, sore muscles. Flu??
3:30 PM				1 oz nuts & raisins	Feeling worse. Going home early
4:30 PM	240(c)	8 ultr 11 reg		Splitpea soup muffin	
5 PM				banana	
8 PM	150(d)			6 oz apple juice	Vomiting
11 PM	100			6 oz apple juice	
2 AM	120				Vomiting
7 AM	150	8 ultr 9 reg		6 oz orange juice	

You have probably already found the reasons for the reaction at 11 A.M. and the high blood sugar levels later. In spite of jogging in the morning, George missed his midmorning snack. It was a mild reaction because the action of the morning regular insulin was almost over. The slightly high test at noon might have been due to rebound from the reaction, but it is probably more likely that the developing illness was responsible. He took an extra unit of regular insulin before lunch, but by the time he tested at 4:30, his blood sugar had climbed to a fairly high level. Knowing that this was due to the physical stress of the flu, he took four extra units of regular before dinner and reduced the amount of carbohydrate eaten by 100 calories. Dinner was vomited by 8:00, so George tested to see how much more food seemed advisable. Blood sugar at 150, with extra regular still working, told him that some more carbohydrate was needed. The rest of the record shows him using frequent tests to stay in relative balance, despite the effects of the flu.

As you work with your own logs, you will gain skill at interpreting the results and understanding the reasons for high tests and reactions. You will also be able to see the effects of the actions you take to bring blood sugar back to normal as you begin the second part of this step.

7a. Learn to vary insulin dosage, diet, and exercise in order to compensate for high or low tests and to deal with changes in routine

The ability you learn in this step is central to improving blood sugar levels while living a life-style with a great deal of flexibility. When you are skilled in varying the ingredients of your regimen, you are able to live with a level of freedom previously associated with lack of control for a diabetic. You can usually bring blood sugar back to normal within a few hours when it is high. You can handle the effects of illness or emotional stress. You can change schedules, diet, and activity and still maintain acceptable readings. By your conscious decisions you are performing the balancing act that used to take place automatically before you had diabetes.

There are two types of changes you will be making on a day-to-day basis: those designed to correct for tests that are too high or too low, and those necessary to prepare for a change in routine. We can offer some general guidelines for making these alterations in regimen, but the feedback from your tests will help you learn exactly how much you should change insulin, food, or exercise to produce a given change in blood sugar level. At first, it is wise to change only one element at a time so you can see what the effect of the change is. Later you will be skilled enough to change more than one.

Use these target levels, or the specific ones you and your physician have agreed upon, to determine need for short-term changes in insulin, diet, or exercise. These target levels can be difficult to achieve even with dedicated effort. You may need to begin with less demanding goals if stress or other factors make it difficult to achieve this level of control. Negotiate a target you have a fair chance of hitting.

A Menu of Adjustments

If blood sugar is too high	Increase insulin (regular)	or	Increase exercise	or	Decrease carbohy-drates
To prepare for extra activity or exercise	Decrease insulin (regular or intermedi-ate)		or		Increase carbohy-drates

Insulin dosage is probably the easiest factor to change to correct for high readings. Extra insulin taken in this way is called supplemental. The general rule of thumb: If you are an adult of average weight, take one unit of additional regular for each 30 mg/dl above 120 that your premeal test shows. (If you are a child, or an adult under 100 pounds, take one unit for each 50 mg/dl above 150.) Thus, if your usual dose of regular is five units before dinner, take seven units to correct for a test of 180, or nine units if the test is 240. If the high test comes at a premeal time when you don't usually take a shot, go ahead and take a supplement, so long as you eat your usual meal. Usually you should not correct for high tests after a meal; wait to see what the next premeal test is.

It is best not to take supplements before going to bed. (When Ernest was a teenager, he woke up in the hospital after trying to balance a hot fudge sundae with a midnight injection of regular insulin. He overestimated the impact of the forbidden treat because blood glucose testing wasn't available then.)

Usually no more than four to five extra units of regular insulin should be taken at one time, even if blood sugar is very high. It is better to bring it down in steps, thus reducing the risk of severe reactions. *Children or lightweight adults should supplement no more than three units at a time.*

Similarly, you can take a supplement of insulin before a feast or other dietary indulgence to keep the excess from driving your blood glucose sky high. Be cautious here and, in general, increase regular only one or two units. Better to have a slightly high reading later than a heavy insulin reaction caused by too large a supplement. Also, be sure not to take the regular more than half an hour before eating, or you may need to ask for dessert before dinner.

Feedback from your blood tests (especially 1-2 hour postmeal tests) will tell you if you need larger or smaller supplements of regular insulin than the ones indicated here. This is a matter that has to be individually tailored.

You can also make small decreases in insulin dose to prepare for a period of exercise more strenuous than you would usually go through at a particular time. Regular should be cut for a shorter exercise period occurring two to three hours after injection. Intermediate insulin should also be reduced if you expect an extended period of exercise such as working in the garden or hiking all day. Approximate reduction should be at the rate of one unit for each thirty minutes of moderate exercise, or one unit for each fifteen minutes of heavy exercise. But do not decrease dose by more than one-third the total you normally would take at that time. Here, too, your test results and reactions will tell you if the reductions need to be smaller or larger for you.

If supplementing your insulin was the only thing you did to keep blood sugar normal, you would soon encounter a serious side effect: You would soon be putting on weight because the blood sugar that used to be spilled into urine would be stored as fat. Extra insulin may be the easiest way to correct for high tests, but it definitely should not be the only one you use if you wish to avoid a steady weight gain.

So, after working with insulin supplements long enough to learn how to use them, start using the other two tools available for bringing down high blood sugar levels: reduction in meal size and exercise. When your test is high, cut back on carbohydrate (especially rapidly absorbed ones like fruit and white potatoes). Try one slice of toast instead of two, and no fruit if your morning blood sugar is between 150 and 200. Then test an hour after the meal and before lunch to see if this change was enough to bring you back on target. Through trial and error, you will soon see how much to cut back to normalize blood sugar and avoid a reaction.

Eating additional food to compensate for planned exercise is a well-established practice. The rule of thumb here is to add 10 to 15 grams of carbohydrate (such as a medium orange, a half-pint of milk, or a half-ounce of raisins) for each thirty to forty-five minutes of moderate activity. If the exercise goes on for a extended period, you may need additional, rapidly absorbed carbohydrates as you go along (dried fruit or juices). Reactions occurring during exercise and a blood test following exercise indicate just how much extra food you need for the kind of activities you engage in.

Exercise itself is the third tool for reducing blood sugar when it is too high. If the fasting test is between 150 and 240 mg/dl, a brisk walk or a half-hour of dancing between insulin injection and breakfast may be enough to bring blood sugar down to normal. There are so many levels of exercise that it doesn't seem wise to set guidelines here. Again, you have the feedback system necessary to find out how the kind of exercise you like works to reduce blood sugar. Test an hour after the meal and see if the result is back within acceptable limits. After a few trials you will know how much of a particular form of activity it takes to reduce blood sugar a given amount.

There is a limit to the usefulness of exercise in lowering blood sugar. In fact, at levels over 300 mg/dl, exercise will actually drive blood sugar still higher and is likely to produce ketones in your blood and urine. When blood sugar is this high, insulin supplements, moderation in diet, or both are the only ways to reduce it. When you find it necessary to deal with tests this high, it is important not to be excessive in treatment. Serious reactions have resulted from too large supplements of insulin and decreases of food intake. It is better to come down in stages, taking no more than four or five extra units of insulin at a time (three units for a child or adult under 100 pounds), and never cutting more than half of any meal. It is a good idea to monitor your results by testing between meals when doing this.

While learning to make these day-to-day alterations in regimen, systematic record keeping will speed the process. On the basis of your logs, you will soon be able to set your own individual prescriptions for making changes. For each 30 mg/dl over 120, either take one extra unit of insulin or eat so many grams less carbohydrate or do so many minutes of moderate activity (using the values you discover work for you). You will gain a very precise ability to prepare for changes and deal with the results of changes after they occur.

Remember, you are an individual and these are only guidelines. You, in collaboration with your physician, now have the tools to tailor these guidelines precisely to yourself. You are a pioneer in a generation of diabetics who for the first time are able to live a flexible life and still keep blood sugar under good control.

Step 8: Have new lab tests done to measure the effect of your new regimen and establish an ongoing regimen

After you have been on the intensive regimen two to three months, your physician will order new hemoglobin A_1c and blood lipid (fats) test and will probably also want to review your daily logs. This information will give an objective mirror of your level of control. With it, you and your doctor will be able to establish any further changes in ongoing regimen that may be needed.

At this point, you will establish how often to continue testing blood glucose and the level of record keeping to maintain. One study found that control suffered if subjects tested fewer than three or four times a day. Some doctors recommend testing each time insulin is taken and at bedtime. Others suggest at least two tests a day, one of them upon arising. One day a week test before every meal and at bedtime. Whatever the recommendations, many of us simply want to go on testing three to four times a day because the feedback is so valuable. Discuss this and the question of records with your physician.

Step 9: Assess your progress and determine what (if anything) is needed to further improve control

You may have made fantastic progress, with most tests within your target range. Or perhaps you have made significant improvements but are still testing higher than you would like. It may be that your tests show relatively little improvement, even though you have devoted yourself to doing everything the intensive regimen calls for. Your blood sugar level may have bounced up and down with frequent insulin reactions. Possibly you have been struggling just to become willing to follow the regimen.

No matter what you have achieved at this point, it is a time to pause reflectively and congratulate yourself. Even if you are still far out of control and fighting desperately against everything you know is good for you, it is time to retreat from the war with yourself. Whether you have much or little to accomplish, take time to define the progress you have made, what you still need to learn, what obstacles are holding you back, and what you can do to overcome them.

Assessing Your Progress
Give Yourself Some Credit

1. No matter what you have achieved so far, the fact that you are still at work earns point for you. If you feel like it, collect a "hanging-in-there" reward and give yourself some special treat.

2. Go through the list of eleven steps that you have been working on (at the beginning of Chapter 5); see which ones you have completed and which ones still need more work. Make sure you haven't missed any. Again, give yourself credit for what you have done and suspend any tendency to blame yourself for what is still to do done. (If you are one of those who was able to gain optimal control quickly, you are fortunate indeed.)

If you choose to make further improvements in control, go through the following checklist and find what you still need to learn.

1. Do you understand your insulin regimen—what type of insulin you are supposed to take at what times and when each of them peaks? If not, review this with your doctor and read the section in Step 6 describing it.

    Do you understand how the different factors determining blood sugar work? If not, go back to Step 3 and review this information.

2. Is your blood glucose testing accurate? If you haven't taken a class or been instructed in the technique, ask your doctor or nurse to help you and review Step 3.

3. Is your life filled with stress, or are you especially sensitive to stress? If so, read Chapter 11, "Living Well With Stress," and consider taking a stress-management class.

4. Are you finding it difficult to regularize diet, activity, or schedule for this learning period? Use Chapter 3 to help you discover the obstacles.

5. Do you understand your diet and follow it? Need some tips? Read Chapter 9, "Living Well With Your Diet." See a dietitian or nutritionist if you need more information.

6. Do you notice any signs of nighttime reactions or Somogyi effect? (See Chapter 8.) Have you tested blood sugar during the night (around 2:00 or 3:00 A.M.) to be sure you are not having reactions?

7. Are there any irregularities or imbalances in endocrine hormones other than insulin? Your doctor can determine whether this is likely and order tests.

8. Is any other physical condition affecting your control? Discuss this with your doctor.

9. Do you have strong doubts that optimal control is worth the work it takes to achieve it?

    Do you believe that the intensive regimen intrudes on your life too much or creates too much inconvenience?

Review the section of Chapter 4 on the benefits of the intensive regimen and look at your answers to the guide to decision making at the end of that chapter.

Do the work in the next step: maintaining motivation.

Do you doubt yourself—either your ability to learn or your worth as a person? See Chapter 14, "Living Well With Yourself."

10. Are your trying to learn the intensive regimen at a time when too many other demands are being made on you? It may be that problems with school, work, family, relationships, or emotional difficulties are competing with your need to manage your diabetes well. If so, can you put any of the other challenges on hold? You may decide now to work with a moderate regimen. (See Chapter 6.)

11. Do you feel you have enough support and guidance from your physician and others?

Let your doctor and the other health professionals know what you need. If your requests are legitimate and they are unwilling to meet them, consider changing doctors. (See Chapter 12, "Living Well With Your Medical Team.")

Have you enlisted the support of other diabetics? (See Chapter 13, "Living Well With Others With Diabetes.")

12. Is there anything else you can think of that could be the reason for your difficulty?

If you feel tempted to throw in the towel because you've had a hard time gaining the level of control you hoped for, you may need a short breather. Back off from the thousand and one details you are trying to master and look at your whole situation. Even if your tests are not yet on target, you may find that you have made important progress in mastering some of the tasks of the intensive regimen. You haven't failed. It's just that there is more to be learned.

You may need to accept a higher blood sugar level while you work on motivation or on reducing your stress level or other issues outside diabetes. Or there may be physical conditions that make control more difficult to attain. You may need to find a physician who is better informed or more in sympathy with your goals.

If, after pinpointing the reasons for your frustration, you decide to put the intensive regimen on the shelf for a while, be kind to yourself. Make a commitment to reopen the subject at a scheduled date in the future. Understand the reasons you have made the decision and let them guide you to your next step in your ongoing diabetes education. Follow the moderate regimen, or at least the loose one, and work on the issues that have stopped you. There may be powerful negative beliefs or self-image issues (see Chapter 14, "Living Well With Yourself") that must be cleared up before you will be willing to accept a gift as valuable as optimal control. Or perhaps there are too many problems outside health that you are dealing with. Whatever the reason, if you discontinue the intensive regimen now without blaming yourself, you will find it much easier to begin again later.

You may also decide, on the basis of this experience with the intensive regimen, that you simply do not choose to manage diabetes at this level. As we have said before, you are the only one who can balance the questions of physical health and quality of life involved in this decision. Living well with diabetes is finding the balance that works for you.

Step 10: Maintain motivation for continuing with the intensive regimen

The intensive regimen becomes easier to manage once you know the basics. The testing schedule is not as demanding; you have the knowledge and skills you need to be fairly flexible in life-style and still maintain good control; and you have created a set of new habits that serve your purpose of living well with diabetes. Your regimen is easier, but it is not what most people would call easy. You have taken a position of responsibility, one calling for day-to-day awareness and decision making. It is advisable to take steps ensuring continuing motivation so that this responsibility does not begin to feel like a burden.

The immediate rewards of following the intensive regimen offer direct reinforcement of motivation. When you have immediate feedback on blood sugar level and the ability to do something about it, you enjoy a sense of power and control. (Anyone who has lived with diabetes for many years knows the frustration and sense of powerlessness that often accompanies attempts to gain control.) This emotional benefit is extended by the feeling of physical well-being that results from optimal control. Don't take these improvements in mind and body for granted. Remember that you have worked hard to achieve them and that you will continue to enjoy them by respecting your regimen.

You can also use the long-term benefits of optimal control as a way of remaining willing to adhere to regimen. You are increasing your chances of living a long and healthful life. Day by day you are maintaining a body that functions more like that of a nondiabetic. If you have children, you are more likely to be a fully active parent throughout their childhood. If you are a woman who wants to become pregnant, you can be more sure of a safe pregnancy and a healthy baby. Periodically review what your personal reasons for living well are, and keep in mind how the intensive regimen will help you get what you want in your life.

Contact with others following the same regimen can also reinforce your motivation. Participation in a support group, or having friends with diabetes you can call on when you need understanding and encouragement, helps in a special way. You are talking with people who really know what you are dealing with. You are able to get practical tips from the old-timers and you yourself are soon giving valuable aid to the beginners. It is easier to stay involved with quality self-care when you know you are not alone.

Earlier we described the role of brief vacations from tight management as a way of lifting the sense of burden. With the skills in varying insulin, diet, and exercise you have learned, you can probably relax your regimen for a day or two, and not end up with severely elevated blood sugar levels. When doing this, it is wise not to set up conditions that might cause severe insulin reactions: too much added regular insulin, late meals, or "meals" of sweets unaccompanied by more slowly absorbed carbohydrates. It is much easier to continue with the intensive regimen if you do not think of it as a straitjacket that labels any departures as cheating. (That's a word we can do without!) Living well includes brief periods of relaxed control as part of the regimen itself.

If at any time you feel a strong resistance to continuing with the intensive regimen, remember that there are steps you can take to explore the causes and deal with them. Be aware of any rationalizations or denials that you use to justify the resistance. Don't accept, "I'm really too busy," or "I don't need to be so careful," "I'm all right now," or "It won't do any good anyway." Use Chapter 3, "Help!" to gain awareness of what is happening and ask for personal help if you need to.

Step 11: Celebrate!

When you finish learning the intensive regimen, you have completed the most demanding set of learning tasks medicine has to offer its patient (and long-suffering) students. Celebrate your accomplishment. Let your family and friends know what it means to you and to them. After all, most of what you are doing to live well with diabetes would help them live more healthful lives, too. Share with them the joy of reaching your goal. It will help you to continue your new level of self-care not to keep it to yourself. You might take this task quite literally and have a party or a special dinner to announce your "graduation." It can be as subtle or as exuberant as fits your style.

If you have chosen to work with a reward system, now is the time to collect whatever external prize you contracted for. In fact, even if you haven't been working with this idea in mind, you might feel like giving yourself something very special, beyond the intrinsic and priceless prize of good control itself. It doesn't have to be a thing to buy. It might be an experience you have been postponing, a kind of relationship you have not felt ready for, or even a quiet time alone, away from all other demands. You will know what is right for you.

Next Steps

You will also know what more you need to learn about diabetes. Mastering the intensive regimen does not mean that you have finished with your diabetes education. Look through the other sections of the book to see what you need to study next. The pace will be much easier and you will be working on the basis of the solid learning that you have just completed.

Fortunately, you are engaged in a lifelong learning process, as there will always be new research and new techniques for diabetes care. Let us hope that the innovative self-care represented in this book is totally outmoded by new breakthroughs in a short time. To keep up with new developments, you can subscribe to such publications as *Diabetes in the News*, published by Ames, *Diabetes Forecast*, published by the American Diabetes Association, or *Diabetes Self-Management*. (See the Appendix at the end of the book for addresses.) If you are willing to wade through medical jargon, two excellent journals, *Diabetes Care* and *Diabetes Spectrum*, are available in medical libraries. Your local ADA chapter is another source of continuing diabetes education.

The Moderate Regimen

LEARNING THE MODERATE REGIMEN

1. Be sure you have a positive setting for your diabetes learning, a physician who agrees with your goals, and support from family, friends, and other people with diabetes.

2. Have lab tests of hemoglobin A_1c and blood lipids (triglycerides and cholesterol) done to indicate your present level of control.

3. Learn the skills and information needed for managing your diabetic control through the moderate regimen.

   a. Learn how to test blood sugar and urine. Understand the meaning of lab tests relevant to control. Know the criteria of control.

   b. Review Chapter 8, on recognizing and treating insulin reactions.

   c. Survey the basics of diabetic metabolism (how your system processes food and liquids to produce energy and growth).

   d. Understand all the different factors that determine blood sugar level.

4. Determine the level of regularity of diet, activity, and schedule you are willing to follow. Establish a schedule of blood and urine testing that is acceptable to you.

5. With your doctor's guidance, establish your ongoing insulin regimen (no more than two injections of insulin per day; use of the insulin pump is not recommended for the moderate regimen). Set target levels for your tests and action to be taken when blood sugar level is high.

6. Observe the variations in blood sugar level caused by stress, illness, changes in food and exercise, and other factors. Learn to vary insulin dosage, diet, and exercise cautiously to compensate for high or low tests and to deal with changes in routine.

7. Have new lab tests done after two or three months to determine the effect of your new regimen.

8. Assess your progress. Find out what you need to do now to obtain further improvements in control or to maintain the level you have achieved. If you have not achieved all of your goals, determine the obstacles and how to overcome them.

9. Take steps to maintain your motivation for continuing to work on improving control.

10. Celebrate!

Step 1: Be sure you have a positive setting for your diabetes learning

There are many different reasons for choosing a moderate level of control. It may be the level that best balances the whole spectrum of needs in your life. For some, following the moderate regimen represents an enormous improvement in management. For others, it is a fall-back position chosen after attempting the intensive regimen and finding too many obstacles in the way. Some will be comfortable with this level of control until their motivation is boosted by an event like the onset of complications. Some will see it as only a temporary treatment plan until they have time and energy for learning the more disciplined approach.

Whatever your reasons for selecting the moderate regimen, it is important that you allow yourself the most basic ingredient of living well—accepting the choice you have made. The intensive regimen is praised so highly that you may feel a bit anxious, perhaps even guilty about choosing "second-best." Feelings like these are not good for your health.

Your decision about the regimen to follow was not made in isolation. You weighed your needs as a person and as a diabetic, your motivation, and the support available to you. The moderate regimen seems to you to be the wisest choice. Live well with it. (We have built into the regimen a periodic review of this choice—Step 8.)

As you work with this regimen, you may find your interest in care of diabetes growing, or other concerns may diminish, allowing you to devote more time to diabetes care. Simply having the immediate feedback of blood glucose testing may improve your control and increase your motivation to manage your diabetes. Gradually you may find yourself moving toward improved control, learning the information and skills needed at the pace that is right for you.

You may feel anxious because you are not ready or willing to gain optimal control right away. Many of us have experienced a degree of anxiety connected with the possibility of developing complications. It was just something we lived with, consciously or unconsciously. It is natural to experience it, and there are positive things you can do to handle it (see Chapter 15).

We cannot yet say with certainty that the intensive regimen reduces the risk of complications. There are strong clues indicating that it will do so, but the results of the best research thus far (the Diabetes Control and Complications Trial) will not be available until 1994. Furthermore, until the last few years, a moderate level of control was the very best one could attain. Past studies indicate that people who managed their diabetes at this moderate level had fewer complications than those whose blood sugar levels were higher. So you can find some reassurance in this: The moderate regimen is likely to reduce your risks, though possibly not as much as the intensive regimen.

All of the suggestions made in Step 1 of the intensive regimen are applicable here, so you can continue by reviewing that information. See what you need to do to be sure you have adequate support: a physician you can work with effectively, family and friends acquainted with your project, and other diabetics with whom you can compare notes. *Go to Chapter 5, Step 1.*

Step 2: Have lab tests done to determine your present level of control

Hemoglobin A_1c and the blood lipids (fats) tests will allow you to see how effective your previous regimen has been. You and your physician can set goals for these tests that are reasonable, given the moderate regimen. Then new lab tests every three months, along with your own feelings of well-being, will be the best cue to how you are doing. You will find that the feedback from the tests will be very helpful, although at first you may need guidance from your doctor in interpreting them. *See Chapter 5, Step 2* of the intensive regimen for details.

Step 3: Learn the skills and information needed for managing your diabetic control through the moderate regimen

3a. Learn how to test blood sugar and urine

A major difference from the intensive regimen emerges in this step. Although you will still be using home blood glucose testing, you will not be doing it as often and you will also be testing for glucose in your urine. (Possibly, one of the reasons you chose a moderate regimen was that you did not want to test your blood several times a day.) The best schedule of testing for this level of control would be to test your blood glucose level before taking your morning insulin and to test your urine before meals and at bedtime. The daily fasting blood sugar test allows you to supplement your morning shot with regular to compensate for high readings when they occur. Starting the day in control helps you stay controlled throughout the day. The later urine tests give a very rough idea of how well you maintain control throughout the day. (Specifically, they tell whether blood sugar is staying over 180 mg/dl or so before meals. More on this later.) You may also find yourself more willing to test your blood a second time than to test your urine at all. If so, fine!

If this is more testing than you are willing to do, determine a minimal schedule of testing that you feel able to follow consistently. Blood tests two or three times a week and urine tests once or twice a day are better than none. Schedule the urine tests at different times each day so you can see the pattern of results throughout the day, before and after meals, when you look at your log for several days.

By starting to test regularly, you will be creating a habit that you can expand on later. Even a few blood tests each week can help you improve control to some extent. Some people find it helpful to make a written contract with themselves or their doctor, stating the number of tests they will do. Then a report is regularly filed with the results.

You should do additional blood glucose tests when illness upsets your control and to check your perception of insulin reactions. Sometimes you may mistake symptoms of anxiety and stress for those of reactions to insulin. If you show any signs of Somogyi reactions during the night, you can find out whether blood sugar is low by testing around 2:00 or 3:00 in the morning. This special form of insulin reaction causes high fasting blood sugar tests that may mistakenly lead to increases in insulin dose. Whenever insulin dosage is more than 35 units a day, and morning blood sugar tests are high, you should check for low blood sugar during the night. It might also be the "dawn phenomenon." (See Chapter 8 for a full discussion of Somogyi reactions.)

It would help to go to a home blood glucose testing class if one is available, or to have your doctor or nurse instruct you in the correct testing procedures. A number of suggestions on home testing are given in Chapter 5, Step 3a. Also, read the previous sections on laboratory tests and record keeping. With the moderate regimen, a different set of target values is necessary for evaluating your blood tests and urine tests than with the intensive program.

Moderate Regimen Target Glucose Levels

Fasting blood sugar test	70-150 mg/dl
Before meal blood sugar test	70-180 mg/dl
1-2 hr after meal blood sugar test	140-250 mg/dl
Before-meal urine test	Negative
Bedtime urine test	Negative or ¹/4%

We need to redeem the value of urine sugar testing. Blood sugar testing has offered such an improvement in accuracy that there is a tendency to dismiss the old urine test. This is a mistake for anyone who has not yet chosen the intensive level of diabetes management. While limited, the traditional test still provides useful information. It tells you if your blood sugar has been higher than about 180 mg/dl (the exact level varies from person to person) since you last urinated. This does not give adequate feedback for optimal control, but it can help you keep to a moderate level of control. If your tests are usually negative, you know that your blood sugar has been below 180 or so.

One of the shortcomings of urine testing is that the sample tested may reflect earlier blood glucose values. It is possible to have a positive test while undergoing an insulin reaction. For this reason, to get a current reading, you should empty your bladder completely and then urinate again in ten or twenty minutes. Testing this second sample gives a more up-to-date reading. (Testing the first sample gives you an idea of how much sugar was spilled during the whole time since you last urinated.)

Another problem with urine tests is that the level at which blood sugar spills into the urine varies from person to person. This level is called the renal threshold. Someone with a low renal threshold will show a positive urine test when the blood sugar is 140 or lower. Another person, with a high threshold, will not have a positive test until blood sugar is 200 or higher. (The average level at which sugar spills into the urine is 160-180 mg/dl.) The renal threshold may change over time, usually becoming higher with age or as kidneys function less well. Pregnancy also affects the renal threshold.

Finding Your Renal Threshold

This variability makes it important for you to determine what your specific blood sugar spilling point is. This knowledge makes urine testing a much more effective tool. You can identify your renal threshold by testing both blood sugar and urine sugar at the same time. Probably the easiest way to do this is to test every thirty to forty-five minutes, beginning when urine sugar is positive and continuing until it is negative. Empty your bladder, test your blood sugar, and then urinate again a few minutes later and test this sample (using Testape, Diastix or the Bm uG urine test, which are more sensitive than tablets.) Drinking a glass of water each time you urinate will help. Record results of both tests until you can see the threshold level. A sample log illustrates this process:

Time A.M.	Blood Sugar Test (mg/dl)	Urine Test (%)
9:00	240	
9:10		2
9:45	200	
9:50		1
10:30	160	
10:35		¼
11:00	140	
11:05		Negative

This person has a low renal threshold. A positive urine test here indicates that blood sugar is over 150. Another example shows a high threshold:

143

Time P.M.	Blood Sugar Test (mg/dl)	Urine Test (%)
6:00	300	
6:05		1
6:45	260	
6:50		$1/4$
7:30	220	
7:35		$1/10$
8:00	200	
8:05		Negative

In the second example, the threshold is somewhere between 200 and 220 mg/dl blood sugar. A negative test indicates only that blood sugar level is less than that; it may be anywhere from very low (40 mg/dl) to fairly high (200 mg/dl) and still be negative.

Of the different products for testing urine, Clinitest tablets give results that are easy to read, but they are less sensitive and harder to use than the strips. Ames Diastix are easy to use, but the color continues to change after the required thirty seconds, so you must read your results quickly. Ames Clinistix show only if urine is positive or negative, with no percentage given. Boehringer Mannheim's uG strips give easy-to-read colors that do not continue changing. You can get a specific reading that shows whether you are negative, a little high, or very high. If your urine is positive, this test has to wait five minutes for a final reading. Tests results can be affected seriously by large doses of vitamin C and some medications. Read the instructions to see if this is true with your product.

A second type of urine test, for urinary ketones, will provide very important feedback on certain occasions. Ketones in your urine indicate that your diabetes is getting out of control due to a relative insufficiency of insulin (too much food, not enough insulin, or too much physical or emotional stress). Both tablets and strips are available; you should know how to use both. (A new home *blood* test strip is now available for testing ketones, called KetoSite. It is manufactured by GDS Diagnostics, in Elkhart, Indiana.) It is especially important to check for ketones if you are ill (even with a bad cold) or experiencing high blood sugars (greater than 240 mg/dl) or 4+ urine sugars. (See end of this book for more information on ketoacidosis.)

3b. Review the chapter on recognizing and treating insulin reactions

Anyone working on improved control of diabetes risks having more insulin reactions while establishing the new level of regimen. Handling reactions may seem like old news to you, but you will find some new approaches in Chapter 8. *Go to Chapter 8.*

3c. Survey the basics of diabetic metabolism

Go to Chapter 5, Step 3c.

3d. Understand all the different factors that determine blood sugar level

The information given on these subjects above will help you gain a general understanding of the ups and downs of your blood sugar level, even though you won't be working intensively to keep it close to normal range at this point. Later, if you decide to move to the intensive regimen, you can review it in more detail.

Go to Chapter 5, Step 3d.

Step 4: Determine the level of regularity of diet, activity, and schedule you are willing to follow

With this step, we have come to one of the contradictions of the moderate regimen. On this treatment plan, you have a wider range of acceptable blood sugar levels than on the intensive program, but you also have less capacity for adapting to irregularities. Without blood tests several times a day to guide you, you are more likely to have reactions or high blood sugar levels if you do not follow a fairly regular diet, activity plan, and schedule. (Some people prefer to keep blood sugar level a bit high to avoid reactions.) The intensive regimen, on the other hand, allows much more flexibility once you are past the first two or three months needed to learn it.

Ideally, your choice of moderate regimen means that you will stick to a fairly consistent healthful meal plan, either using exchanges or calorie count, with times of meals scheduled fairly closely (not more than an hour off schedule unless you know your blood sugar is high). When a meal must be delayed, you can eat a snack and deduct the calories or exchanges from the meal. Similarly, physical activities should be fairly regular from day to day, with adjustments in insulin dosage or food when there is an increase or decrease in the amount of exercise. As you gain experience with such adjustments, you may find it possible to increase the flexibility of this regimen.

It is up to you to decide just how regular you are willing to be in your management of diabetes. Fortunately, the combination of your home blood and urine tests and the hemoglobin A_1c test in the lab will tell you if your decision allows you to maintain a moderate level of control over a two- or three-month period. If the hemoglobin test is too high, you will know that you need greater regularity. Work with your doctor to find the places where your regimen needs to be tightened up.

Step 5: With your doctor's guidance, establish your ongoing insulin regimen

Your insulin regimen is the overall dosage of one or two types of insulin taken in a single morning injection, or a dose split between morning and predinner injections. To work with it well, you need to know the pattern of insulin activity—when it begins, when it peaks, and how long it is effective. Four insulin plans are available for the moderate regimen. (We do not recommend that people on the moderate regimen use more than two injections a day, nor should they use the insulin pump. These more intensive regimens require more frequent blood sugar tests and a stricter control program to be effective and safe.)

Moderate Insulin Regimens

Plan 1: A single daily dose of intermediate-acting insulin (NPH or Lente), taken 20 to 60 minutes before the first meal of the day.

Plan 2: A single daily dose of intermediate and rapid-acting (regular or Semilente) insulin mixed, taken 20 to 60 minutes before the first meal.

Plan 3: A split dose of intermediate-acting insulin, part taken before breakfast, part before dinner.

Plan 4: A split dose mixing intermediate- and rapid-acting insulins before breakfast and dinner.

Plan 1

The single daily shot of NPH or Lente insulin was the standard insulin regimen for many years. This was a convenient breakthrough in the beginning, compared to the earlier multiple-dose plans using regular alone. Only one injection a day! It must have felt like an enormous improvement, especially since we had only urine testing to show how well controlled we were each day.

Unfortunately, for most insulin-dependent diabetics, convenience is the only strength of this regimen. One shot of intermediate insulin has an extended peak, usually not beginning until the afternoon and lasting through early evening. (Thus, morning high blood sugar levels and afternoon reactions are common.) By evening, the insulin action is waning and often there is insufficient insulin to prevent high blood sugar levels overnight. Since there is only one long peak of activity, it is difficult for you to make adjustments to keep your tests within the moderate target range. Probably only a person whose pancreas still produces a substantial amount of insulin can maintain a moderate level of control on this treatment plan. A single dose of long-acting Ultralente insulin may also work for you. See Chapter 5, p. 114 for Gary's Ultralente anecdote. Gary is a strong proponent of using Ultralente, either as a "basal" insulin or in the single dose regimen if the circumstances fit.

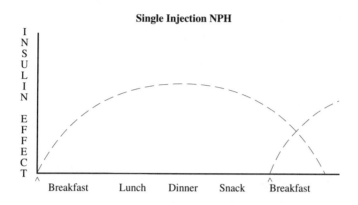

Single Injection NPH

Plan 2

The single injection here mixes rapid-acting insulin with intermediate to cover the need for insulin during the time between breakfast and lunch. The regular dosage can be increased to reduce high blood sugar or reduced if there will be added exercise in the morning. Morning control is improved, but care must still be exercised to avoid afternoon reactions. With most people, it is still likely that blood sugar will rise during the night.

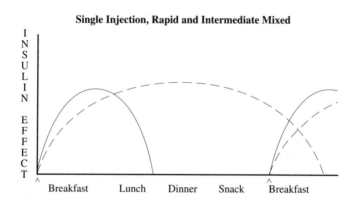

Single Injection, Rapid and Intermediate Mixed

Plan 3

With intermediate insulin (NPH or Lente) taken twice a day, there is a better overall distribution of insulin activity, with peaks in the early afternoon and around bedtime. Overnight coverage is improved, and you are more likely to arise with blood sugar within your target range. Small doses of regular can be added to the intermediate when tests show high blood sugar. Since each of the NPH injections is smaller, the effective duration of action is shorter. The overlap between the two shots helps to handle the mealtime insulin need following breakfast and dinner.

If one is taking two shots of insulin a day, anyway, Plan 4 provides much better coverage and flexibility.

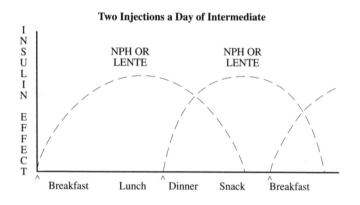

Plan 4

Two injections of rapid- and intermediate-acting insulin, one before breakfast and one before dinner, provide the most effective distribution of insulin activity available under the moderate regimen.

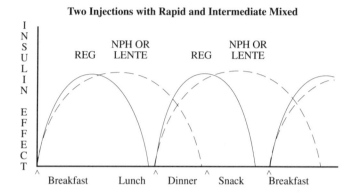

Two Injections with Rapid and Intermediate Mixed

With this plan, a peak of insulin activity follows each meal and an adequate supply continues through the night. (The same schedule is used in the intensive regimen. Combined with frequent blood glucose testing, it allows normal or near-normal blood sugar levels for some.) It is possible for you to learn to vary the amounts of either kind of insulin cautiously to prepare for changes in routine and to vary the regular to correct the high blood sugar levels. In this way you gain more flexibility than the other moderate insulin regimens offer.

These four insulin regimens are described in terms of idealized patterns of insulin activity. In any specific case, each type of insulin may have a pattern of activity that is very different from the averages. This is the reason you will be working closely with your physician at this stage, identifying the pattern at work in your case by studying your test logs. Your physician may recommend a variation on one of these plans, or even a plan not mentioned, to give you insulin activity that will match your life style and physical needs.

Step 6: Observe the variations in blood sugar level caused by stress, illness, changes in food and exercise, and other factors

Earlier you studied the different influences on blood sugar level—insulin, diet, exercise, and physical and emotional stress. Now you can apply that information to understand your daily and weekly diabetes records. Seeing your blood or urine glucose levels swinging up and

150

down and not knowing why they change can be very frustrating. But if you keep thorough records for a few weeks, you can quickly learn to read the reasons for your fluctuations. With understanding, you gain more power to control your blood sugar levels.

We will illustrate this process by looking at several sample logs of people on the moderate regimen.

Daily Diabetes Log

Bill takes two shots of NPH insulin daily, twenty units before breakfast and twelve units before dinner. He records only carbohydrates under the "Food" heading and usually eats snacks midmorning, in the afternoon, and at bedtime. His urine tests begin to show sugar when his blood sugar is around 200 mg/dl.

DATE & TIME	BLOOD OR URINE TEST & REAC- TIONS	INSULIN DOSAGE	ACTIVITY & EXERCISE	FOOD	COMMENTS: Stress, illness, etc.
5-12 7 AM	150 mg/dl	20 NPH	30 min bike	2 toast grape- fruit	
11 AM	strong react. (a)			roll of hard candies	
12 noon	2% urine gl (b)			cut 1 bread & fruit	
3 PM	1%			cut snack (c)	
5:30 PM	neg	12 NPH		normal din	
8 PM					Big fight with Sue. She yelled. I bit my tongue.
10 PM	300 mg/dl (d)			no snack	

DATE & TIME	BLOOD OR URINE TEST & REAC- TIONS	INSULIN DOSAGE	ACTIVITY & EXERCISE	FOOD	COMMENTS: Stress, illness, etc.
5-13, 7 AM	180 (e)	20 NPH	30 min bike	2 toast	
10 AM				crackers	
12 noon	neg			normal lunch	
3 PM					
5 PM	neg			nuts & raisins	Knew dinner would be be late
7:30 PM	1% (f)	12 NPH		Mexican din	Extra carbos & 2 beers
10 PM	150				
5-14 7 AM		20 NPH		usual brkf	

First, go through this log and explain the blood or urine sugar readings or reactions followed by a letter (a-f). Then read the following paragraphs.

Bill's reaction at 11:00 A.M. (a) on May 12 occurred because he missed his midmorning snack, which was especially important given the bike ride earlier.

The strength of the reaction caused him to overtreat it with a whole pack of hard candies. This, plus blood sugar rebound caused by the stress of the reaction, produced a 2 percent urine glucose test at noon (b). Since he starts spilling sugar into his urine only at 200 mg/dl, the 2 percent reading means blood sugar may have been as high as 300 mg/dl. He reduced carbohydrates at lunch to compensate and elimi- nated his snack (c) when urine still tested positively at 3:00. His urine test before dinner was negative (which only shows that it was under 200 mg/dl) but the upsetting fight with his girlfriend caused another blood sugar peak by bedtime (d). He used a blood sugar test when he normally would have tested urine so he could see the impact of the strong emotional stress. He eliminated his evening snack.

His fasting blood test the next morning (e) was down to 180 mg/dl, 30 above his target range for fasting tests, so he omitted fruit from breakfast and made his bike ride more energetic than usual to compensate. (Note: A urine test would have been negative for him because of his slightly high renal threshold.)

These changes in diet and activity balanced blood sugar enough that urine tests were negative at lunch and at 5:00 P.M. Knowing that dinner would be late, he ate an extra snack to avoid reactions. Bill over ate at dinner, which produced a 1 percent urine test at 10:00 (f). This would probably indicate that his blood sugar was over 240. By omitting his late night snack on the basis of this test, he was able to return to his target range for fasting tests by the next morning.

Daily Diabetes Log

Sandra, a working mother with two children, takes 40 units of NPH before breakfast. She records only carbohydrates in the food column and usually snacks in the afternoon and before bed. Her urine tests begin to show sugar when her blood sugar is around 160 mg/dl.

DATE & TIME	BLOOD OR URINE TEST & REACTIONS	INSULIN DOSAGE	ACTIVITY & EXERCISE	FOOD	COMMENTS: Stress, illness, etc.
2-5, 6:30 AM	180 mg/dl	40 NPH		cut 1 bread no fruit (a)	Kids wild!
11:30 AM	reaction (b)		missed jazz dance class	2 donuts	Too much, but I've got to be sharp for noon meeting
12:15 PM				2 rolls bean soup 1/2 piece choc cake	Client insisted I share cake
3:00 PM	peeing a lot! (c) thirsty			skip snack	Must be high

153

DATE & TIME	BLOOD OR URINE TEST & REAC- TIONS	INSULIN DOSAGE	ACTIVITY & EXERCISE	FOOD	COMMENTS: Stress, illness, etc.
5:30 PM	4+ urine 1+ ketones (d)		took kids for 40 min walk	raw veggie salad & broth	
9:30 PM	still peeing xtra (e)			skipped snack	
2-6 6:30 AM	4+ urine but 150 mg/dl	40 NPH (f)		2 toast, 1/2 orange	

Again, see how you explain the test results and symptoms marked by a letter (a-f), and then read the following.

By cutting too much carbohydrate at breakfast (a), Sandra found herself with low blood sugar before lunch (b). Lunch was an important meeting with a business client, so she knowingly overtreated the insulin reaction to be sure she wouldn't have another one. Too many doughnuts, a usual amount of lunch, a missed exercise period, and the stress of the meeting conspired to increase her blood sugar to a symptomatic level (c) and (d). She knew from the excess urination and thirst that her blood sugar was fairly high, so she skipped her afternoon snack, and finding ketones in her urine, ate a very light dinner. Sandra's blood sugar stayed high in spite of reduced carbohydrates and an evening walk with the kids (e). (Remember, when blood sugar is high, each unit of insulin is less effective at lowering it, and exercise may even cause it to increase.) Using frequent urination as her feedback, she skipped her bedtime snack. Her morning urine test was high (reflecting earlier high blood sugar), but her blood sugar test indicated she was within her target range (f). By cutting back on food, she had been able to cut the high blood sugar down to size.

Learn to vary insulin dosage, diet, and exercise cautiously to compensate for high or low tests and to deal with changes in routine.

Begin this step by reviewing Chapter 5, Step 7b. The basic kinds of changes you can make are described there, although the amount of change advised is for the person on that regimen only. With fewer blood sugar tests to guide changes, you will have to work much more cautiously. After you read that material, come back to this point.

Supplementary insulin can be used when tests are high or to prepare for a larger-than-usual meal. Supplements are always taken as regular insulin so the impact is over a limited period of time. Do not take extra insulin on the basis of tests of urine that has been in your bladder for more than fifteen or twenty minutes. (It may represent high blood sugar levels from hours ago.) Use urine samples collected a few minutes after you have completely emptied your bladder. Also, take into account what you have discovered about your renal threshold, the level at which you spill glucose from bloodstream into urine. If you have done the tests comparing urine and blood sugar readings described above under "Finding Your Renal Threshold" (Step 3a in this chapter), you will have a better idea of what your urine tests actually mean.

You can make such supplements of insulin more accurate (and safer) if you usually base them on blood sugar tests rather than urine tests. More and more people on the moderate regimen are using blood sugar tests when they feel a need to, even though they use urine tests on a daily basis.

When your blood sugar control is upset by physical illness, emotional stress, or other factors, you may want to do more blood sugar tests than usual. The greater accuracy will help you deal with the unusual conditions.

A rule of thumb for supplementing insulin on the basis of urine tests is to use 5 percent of your daily dose if the reaction is 1-2 percent, and 10 percent of your daily dose if the reading is over 2 percent.

Urine Test (%)	Daily Total Dose	Extra Regular Units to Take	% of Total Dose
1-2	20	1	5
2+	20	2	10
1-2	50	2-3	5
2-5	50	5	10

If your supplement is based on a blood sugar test, take one unit of regular for every 30 mg/dl over 120 your test shows, up to five units. It is wise not to take more than five extra units of regular at a time (2-3 units if you are a child or small adult). If your blood sugar level is still high at the next test, you can take another supplement then. Avoid taking supplemental insulin at bedtime unless your doctor advises it because of severe illness and very high blood sugar.

If you are consistently spilling sugar into your urine (more than one test a day or even one test at the same time every day), you should discuss this with your doctor. You may need a larger standard dose of insulin or an adjustment in your diet.

Supplements of regular insulin can also be taken before a special meal that you know will be larger or richer than usual. How much extra to take depends, of course, on the size of the meal. At first, don't take more than one or two units extra and see what your next test is. By trial and error, you will learn how much to add, but it is better to err by adding too little than too much. Be sure not to take the supplement too early. Special meals have a way of being delayed.

When you are planning to be more active than usual, you can compensate by taking less insulin or eating more. If you take only NPH, reduce insulin only if the extra activity will last for an hour or more, or if you know it will be occurring around the time of your insulin peak (roughly 6-12 hours after injections). Otherwise it is better to eat extra food to cover the exercise period. Generally one extra serving of carbohydrate (a slice of bread, for instance) should be eaten for every 30 minutes of hard exercise.

Do not rely on increases in insulin only to correct for high blood or urine sugar tests. You should also bring blood sugar down by adjusting exercise and food. This is especially important in the moderate regimen, because you are likely to have more high blood sugar levels than the person on the intensive plan. If you use only insulin supplements to reduce these highs you will gain weight.

Remember that when blood sugar is quite high (over 250 or 300), exercise is not likely to lower it and may even cause an increase. Meals may be reduced by one or two carbohydrate servings, but you should not fast because of the risk of severe reactions if there is no food in your intestines. The safest way of reducing a very high blood sugar level is to take a series of small injections of regular (10% of daily dose), four to six hours apart until urine tests show less than 1 percent glucose or until blood sugar tests are under 200 mg/dl. (Someone with a total daily dose of 40 units should take no more than four units at a time.) When you are lowering an extra-high blood sugar level in this way, it is wise to rely on the greater precision of the blood glucose tests to guide you. Urine tests can still be positive when blood sugar has already reached normal range. If you have high blood sugar and ketones in your urine or are ill, you probably should contact your physician for guidance.

Step 7: Have new lab tests done after two or three months to determine the effect of your new regimen

At this point, you will have solid feedback on the effectiveness of your regimen. Tests for hemoglobin A_1c and blood lipids, together with your home test records, will let you know if you have found the right balance in your program of self-care. As you review the results with your physician, take an objective point of view. You have certain target levels you want to achieve. If you haven't reached them, suspend all judgments on yourself and simply look for the reasons. The next step will help you do this.

Step 8: Assess your progress and determine what (if anything) is needed to improve control further

Again, you can use the parallel step in the intensive regimen, with just a few changes. Where it refers to the eleven steps in the intensive, go to the beginning of this chapter instead, where the steps of the moderate learning process are listed. And, of course, substitute the word *moderate* for *intensive* throughout. *Go to Chapter 5, Step 9.*

If you find that you have learned all you need to manage well at a moderate level of control, we suggest you take a moment to review the decision you made at the beginning. When you consider all factors, is a moderate regimen still your choice? You may feel content with the improvements in control you have achieved and prefer to give attention to other aspects of your life.

Or you may choose to move on to the intensive regimen. If so, you have already studied a major portion of what you need to learn, so it will be much easier to make the transition. Probably the main changes will be testing blood more frequently, possibly changing insulin regimen, and giving more attention to compensating for the variations you observe. Discuss the necessary changes with your doctor and review each step of the intensive regimen.

Step 9: Maintain motivation for continuing to work on improving control

If you choose to continue managing your diabetes at the moderate level, or if you still have more to learn about this level, keeping your motivation high is important. It may have been an easy process so far, or it may have been intensely frustrating. Either way, you will need to take steps to ensure that you remain willing to continue.

Rereading Step 1 at the beginning of this chapter may be useful. All of the things said about building a positive foundation for this work continue to be relevant now. You might find elements you neglected the first time around but now feel like putting into effect.

Support from other people with diabetes working on improving control is one of the most important ways of keeping motivation strong. If you have not yet found ways of obtaining this, it may be time to do so. Support groups or individual contacts can give valuable emotional support and encouragement. You can receive practical guidance from people who have overcome many of the obstacles you may still be struggling with. You may also be able to help others with problems you have already solved. Serving someone else in this way keeps your motivation high. (See Chapter 13, "Living Well With Other Diabetics.")

Living on a regimen is easier if you do not feel you are in a regiment on active duty every day of the year. Occasional leaves or vacations should be part of your regimen; don't feel that you are cheating at these times. A day or two of relaxed management can make it much easier for you to continue with your usual level of control. If you take supplements of regular insulin to handle any feasts, keep them moderate to avoid severe reactions. (Such vacations are not advisable if you have any infection or a complication that could be made worse by higher blood sugar levels.)

If you have made significant improvement in control, you are probably feeling better, both physically and mentally. This immediate payoff makes it easier for you to continue following your regimen. It also becomes an inspiration for continued learning. This is reinforced by the blood glucose level is and do something about it, you gain power over diabetes, instead of feeling controlled by it. It is natural to want to extend this sense of power by learning more about managing your condition well.

If you feel at any time a strong resistance to continuing with your regimen, remember that there are steps you can take to explore the causes and neutralize them. Be aware of any rationalizations or denials that you use to justify the resistance. Don't accept "I'm really too busy" or "I don't need to be so careful, I'm all right now," or "It won't do any good anyway." Use the help processes in Chapter 3 to gain awareness of what is happening and ask for personal help if needed.

Step 10: Celebrate!

When you finish learning the moderate regimen, you have completed a challenging assignment. You may feel like honoring yourself for your achievement, personally or even publicly, with a party, a dinner, or a picnic. Whether you invite a small group or a large one, give yourself credit for the many things you have learned. What you are doing to live well with diabetes can be generalized. Other than taking insulin and testing blood, the basics of your regimen would give good health to anyone. So share the health.

Now is the time to collect a reward if you promised yourself one to build motivation at the beginning. In fact, even if you didn't make that agreement with yourself then, you might feel you deserve some special thing, event, or experience now. Living well is its own reward, but there is nothing wrong with bonuses from time to time.

Next Steps

You may have chosen to stay at a moderate level of control while you deal with other aspects of having diabetes. Review the Table of Contents to see what else you would like to work on now. You may find that you have learned enough to continue gradually improving your blood sugar management while you focus on other issues.

Possibly, there are problems or challenges in your life that you need to handle while you take an intermission in your diabetes learning (perhaps applying in other areas what you have learned about yourself here). If so, make a date with yourself to reopen the subject in three months or so. Mark the calendar: TIME TO START LEARNING MORE ABOUT DIABETES? Diabetes is a lifelong companion, so you will benefit from also seeing it as a lifelong teacher.

On the other hand, now that you have mastered the moderate regimen, you may be eager to go right on to the intensive program. You have a solid foundation in what you have learned up to now, so it will be much easier than it would have been a few months ago.

(Whatever your next steps, you might consider a subscription to the publications *Diabetes Forecast,* published by the American Diabetes Association, *Diabetes in the News,* published by Ames, or *Diabetes Self-Management.* They are good sources for news on the latest developments in diabetes research and care. See resources in the Appendix.)

The Loose Regimen

"It sure would have helped if someone had told me I was in control, even though my diabetes was out of control. I never saw that I was the one who went on binges or 'forgot' my shot. It just happened, like somebody else was doing it to me."

—*Ernest*

LEARNING THE LOOSE REGIMEN

1. Review the survival issues at the end of the book—insulin reactions, diabetic coma, and infections.

2. Learn to do home blood and urine glucose testing. Do tests occasionally, especially when you are ill or have an infection. Do urine ketone tests when you are ill or experiencing high stress.

3. Take one or two insulin injections daily. (More injections or the insulin pump are not recommended without regular blood sugar testing.)

4. Eat a healthful diet, usually with moderation. Learn how to

161

increase the pleasure of eating without increasing the sugar and fat content.

5. Observe great caution in adjusting insulin dosage.

6. Make a commitment to continuing diabetes learning, maintaining your motivation, and reviewing obstacles to improving control.

The basic belief we assume in this book is that all people who have diabetes are on a controlled regimen, no matter how wildly their blood sugar levels rise and fall. Consciously or unconsciously, you make a series of self-care choices each day. Taken together, they are the regimen you live by. Not taking insulin, missing meals, overeating, keeping an irregular schedule—there are many possible ingredients in the regimens that are usually considered rebellion against any treatment plan.

We prefer to acknowledge the power that you wield if you are at this level of management. If you accept that you do, in fact, control the choices you make, you are more likely to realize that you can make other choices. You can live well while you find ways of using your power to adopt an approach more in tune with your physical needs as a person with diabetes.

So we have outlined a loose regimen, with recommendations for certain minimal self-care standards. It is a fairly simple approach without elaborate lists of tasks. We go to the heart of our philosophy of diabetes care here. This regimen is far from the standards of control recommended for diabetes today. But you can still live well by doing what you can (or will) and not condemning yourself for what you can't (or won't) do. You can live well by finding whatever it is you are willing to do to begin improving control and making a start.

Step 1. Review the survival issues at the end of the book

The highest priority in your diabetes education goes to these three life-or-death issues: insulin reactions, diabetic coma, and infections. Ignorance of these could cost you your life.

If you have insulin reactions often (more than a couple of times a week), you may need more information on avoiding them. Chapter 8, on reactions, could be a lifesaver for you.

Step 2. Learn to do home blood and urine glucose testing

We would also like to suggest that one of your early actions be learning to do home blood glucose tests. Even if you use this skill infrequently, it is one of the most valuable things you can learn. As few as two tests a week have proven effective in helping people with diabetes improve their metabolic control. Keep the test strips available so you can easily test when you want to know how changes in diet, activity, or stress have affected your blood sugar level. If you think your blood sugar becomes high, check it and validate your perception. When you become ill, home blood testing makes it much easier to keep blood sugar from skyrocketing. This can hasten your recovery.

If you wish to learn more about home blood testing, go to Chapter 5, Step 3a. You may find it useful to take a class or ask your doctor or nurse to show you test techniques.

If you have not been doing urine glucose testing, you might also consider this as part of your regimen. Although not particularly useful in the intensive regimen, urine tests still give useful feedback with the less strict treatment plans. You can tell if your blood sugar is more or less controlled, and when it is quite high, you can take cautious action to bring it down.

The test for ketones in the urine is especially important because it indicates when your control is significantly off, because of physical illness or emotional stress or very high blood sugar levels. Information on making the feedback from urine tests more meaningful is in Chapter 6, Step 3a.

Step 3. Take one or two insulin injections daily

(More injections or the insulin pump are not recommended without blood sugar testing.)

Without frequent blood sugar testing, you should not take more than one or two injections of insulin a day. Your physician will help you determine the types of insulin and dosage that will best suit your schedule. Chapter 6, Step 5 describes several one or two injection schedules.

Step 4. Eat a healthful diet, usually in moderation

If you overeat, binge eat and generally ignore your diet, you might find reading Chapter 9 on nutrition rewarding. It contains tips on ways to enjoy food while eating more healthfully.

Step 5. Observe great caution in adjusting insulin dosage

Be cautious in adjusting insulin dosage to compensate for changes in diet and level of activity. You need the feedback of regular blood sugar and urine tests to do this safely. If blood sugar is high because you are ill, consult with your doctor on any changes in the amount of insulin you take.

Step 6. Make a commitment to continuing diabetes learning, maintaining your motivation and reviewing obstacles to improving control

Explore what commitment you are prepared to make to continuing learning about diabetes self-care. Determine for yourself the aspects of diabetes management that you can willing choose to work on. By proceeding in this way, you are likely to learn much faster.

Scan the sections of the moderate and intensive regimens and see if you are attracted to learning about any of this material. And look again through the Table of Contents. Find what you are willing to learn about now. A conversation with your physician or nurse-practitioner might help you define your next steps.

Who Chooses the Loose Regimen?

A variety of people may choose this level of diabetes management.

The loose regimen may be your choice if you are someone:

- Whose life is in turmoil or filled with external demands.

- Who values quality of life-style in the present over the possible reduction of future risks.

- Who feels rebellious and unwilling, or weak and unable to change.

- Who has a poor self-image.

- Who has little money and cannot afford necessary supplies.

We can offer specific guidance to people in each of these groups.

1. If your life is filled with external demands or is in turmoil, set aside some minimum amount of time for learning to manage your diabetes better. As little as ten or twenty minutes a day can be a good beginning. The important thing is making a commitment in spite of a challenging schedule or an overwhelming set of problems. Once you've made a beginning or small first step, it may be easier for you to give diabetes care a higher priority and give more time to it. You may find that some of those other tasks can be scaled down or put on hold for a while. If not, you will still be gradually learning information and skills vital to your well-being.

2. If you have chosen the loose regimen because you tend to live for the moment, valuing present pleasures over future risks, you may be surprised. Many people following more intensive regimens report no shortage of totally enjoyable experiences. For them, greater control is equal to greater freedom. Regular blood glucose testing and the ability to easily adjust insulin, diet, and exercise allow great flexibility in life style, at a relatively small cost in time. This freedom in living carries with it less anxiety about the future. The person who is actively controlling diabetes is doing the best he or she can to reduce the risk of complications later. Physically, you will certainly feel much better when your blood sugar is closer to normal.

    You might find it useful to review the leading pleasures in your life and ask yourself how they can be reconciled with improved diabetes care. There are relatively few absolute contradictions, so long as you are not attached to excess itself as a pleasure. It might help you to talk with others who are following more intensive regimens but who have found ways to respect the pleasure principle.

Although you may feel rock-hard in your habits, you should remember that human beings are actually very adaptable. You can probably think of changes that have occurred in your own life that at first seemed very negative but soon proved to be definite improvements.

3. If rebelliousness or a sense of weakness and incapacity is your style, you may want to work on issues of power. Diabetes regimens are followed with greater ease when you find the source of authority within yourself, rather than in the medical system. You are the one who ultimately decides what you will or will not do, no matter what your doctor says. If you see doctors as authorities who give orders, and then you automatically do the opposite, your rebellion is hardly freedom. If, on the other hand, you feel weak and unable to do what your doctor says, this is often only a covert form of rebellion. Either way you lose.

    Real freedom and power come from consciously deciding what you will do in each situation you face and then leaving these automatic reactions behind. Even if your doctor does tend to give commands, hear them as intelligent advice. Make a conscious choice of what you will or will not do and give yourself room to make new choice. (See Chapters 3 and 14.)

4. Some of us feel that we don't deserve first-class care. "Why bother with me? I'm not worth it." If this is your reason for choosing a relatively casual approach to regimen, you may need to work on developing a more positive self-image. Unfortunately, negative beliefs about yourself tend to produce behavior that confirms them. Escape from this cycle can take place through work on the beliefs themselves or on the behavior. In some cases the assistance of a trained therapist is advisable, but many people have made changes at this level solely through

their own efforts. (See the sections on self-image and beliefs on Chapter 14, "Living Well With Yourself." Chapter 3 also contains techniques you may find helpful.)

5. If you lack the money for home blood glucose testing or other diabetes care supplies, you may be able to gain guidance from your local American Diabetes Association chapter. You may find a staff person there who can help you search for community resources that provide essential supplies. Some health insurance now covers testing supplies and equipment as well as diabetes education. (See the Appendix for discount mail-order supply houses offering significant savings.)

Living Well With Insulin Reactions

"There's nothing makes me feel more anxious than the idea that I may just lose it if I don't eat enough or if I jog too far. I've had one reaction I didn't wake up from and one where I got so confused I forgot I was looking for food. My son finally came home and had to tell me what to do. I don't ever want to go through that again!"

—Jan, a 35-year-old woman

When psychologists ask us what bothers us about having diabetes, we usually cite insulin reactions as our top concern. When we don't respond adequately to this short-term complication of diabetes, we may find ourselves in an embarrassing situation because of things we did in a less-than-coherent state. We may even find ourselves waking up in the hospital or in jail. It's distressingly simple: A very low blood sugar level results in unclear thinking and emotional outbursts. If blood sugar falls too far, we can lose consciousness. No wonder we feel bothered by that one!

Because proper response to insulin reactions is such a vital part of living well with diabetes, this chapter reviews the traditional ways of treating these reactions. And we have added some new approaches to help people change some emotional and behavioral patterns that may cause frequent insulin reactions. There is also a section for the person working with optimal control, since hypoglycemia (low blood sugar) tends to work differently when blood sugar levels are usually near normal than when they are usually high. During the time when you are gaining optimal control, the risk of having reactions is higher than usual, and you need to know what to expect. This is true for people on the insulin pump as well as for those on multiple-injection regimens.

THE ACTION OF REACTION

When blood sugar falls below a certain point (usually around 60-70 mg/dl) our body signals red alert. The resulting stress reaction is to pump out adrenal hormones that produce the racing pulse, thumping heart, nervous feelings, and sweating indicative of a strong insulin reaction. This dramatic response is appropriate, because the situation is a serious one. If our blood sugar level goes too low, we lose consciousness. If it stays too low for too long, we risk brain damage. Our bodies usually respond to the crisis if we do lose consciousness. One of the hormones released in a serious reaction is glucagon, a substance stored in the liver that helps raise blood sugar level. However, repeated insulin reactions can lower the amount of glucagon or glucose available to deal with hypoglycemia.

(The high blood sugar level that may follow a moderate to severe reaction is often caused by the glucagon stimulating more glucose release than is necessary. This is known as the *rebound from a reaction.* The effect is multiplied when the person with diabetes also eats more food than is necessary. More about this rebound effect later in the chapter under "Somogyi Reactions.")

Insulin reactions may be caused by several different factors: a delayed meal or missed snack; an unexpected period of strenuous activity; too much insulin because of a mistake in measuring dosage; a period of strong emotional expression; even a time of relaxation after a week of high tension. In general, it's a matter of food too little or too late, or an excess of activity, insulin or particular kinds of emotional stress.

170

(Stress may lower or raise blood sugar, depending on the circumstances.)

This is really a matter of balance between the different factors affecting blood sugar level. Reactions occur because food, exercise, insulin and possibly the results of stress are out of balance. As we learn to alter these factors, we learn to avoid reactions. We discover how different activities affect blood sugar and how to adjust food intake or insulin dosage to compensate for increased activity. We learn what kind of stress is likely to lower blood sugar for us and when to compensate.

Symptoms of Hypoglycemia

The symptoms of an insulin reaction vary from person to person and from reaction to reaction. Fortunately, home blood glucose testing provides one sure sign: If blood glucose is below 60 to 70 mg/dl, it's time to eat a snack that will be rapidly absorbed. Testing whenever a reaction is suspected or anticipated is excellent practice for the person new to diabetes as well as for the experienced diabetic who is tightening metabolic control. The objective feedback of the test helps you to develop and sharpen awareness of the particular set of symptoms signaling the onset of a reaction for *you*.

Other than blood sugar level itself, the particular symptoms of a reaction depend upon the severity of the reaction, the rapidity of onset, and other individual factors. The classic symptoms of a mild to moderate reaction include lightheadedness, dizziness, shakiness, sweating, increase in pulse rate, and hunger. As the reaction progresses, vision may become blurry and the mind fuzzy. There may be mental confusion, emotional outbursts, or extreme anxiety. A person may forget that he or she is looking for candy or become distracted by the search for the perfect candy bar. (If it's a nocturnal reaction, the person may dream or imagine that the candy has been eaten.) In some cases, a diabetic may even become angry or resistant if anyone else suggests eating something sweet.

Finally, if no food is taken, the diabetic loses consciousness and may experience convulsions. (The muscular movements may be imagined as the body's attempt to squeeze out any sugar the muscles might be storing.) If someone else knows what is happening, treatment can usually revive the person on the spot. Otherwise, it's time for the medic or the emergency room.

This sequence isn't always the same. Sometimes a reaction will approach very quietly, especially if the fall in blood sugar has been very slow. The first sign may be confusion or irritability. There may simply be a sense of unease or difficulty getting to sleep. Or in a time otherwise marked by anxiety or high stress, it may be difficult to notice that a particular bit of shakiness is indicating a reaction rather than more of the old stress. It is important that you know *your* reaction symptoms and variations in them that are likely to occur. Later we will describe ways of increasing your sensitivity to these signs so that you can treat reactions early.

Symptoms of Insulin Reactions

You will experience some, but not necessarily all, of these symptoms, and you may find a few unique to your own body.

- A *mild reaction*—Tiredness or weakness, hunger, sweatiness, chills, cold hands, increased pulse rate, shakiness (or shaky feeling), dizziness, lightheadedness, headache, pallor, difficulty getting to sleep.

- A *moderate reaction*—An increase in any of the above, anxiety, confusion, anger, unclear thinking, loss of emotional control, strange behavior, poor coordination, speech difficulties, blurred, spotty or double vision.

- A *severe reaction*—Stupor, loss of consciousness, convulsions.

Both you and the people close to you should be familiar with these symptoms.

Some people with diabetes do not experience the usual reaction symptoms. Because of reduced production of the hormones that set off the alarm, blood sugar may fall very low, with little or no sign that it is happening. If you suspect that you are not experiencing the usual symptoms of a reaction, discuss this with your physician. Lab tests can determine if you have this type of hormonal lack. "Hypoglycemic unawareness" is being recognized more often, and its causes appear to be more numerous and complex than previously thought. (If you have developed diabetic neuropathy or are taking prescription drugs like beta blockers, you may also not be experiencing some of the typical symptoms such as rapid pulse, shakiness, or sweatiness.)

To a large extent, the symptoms of an insulin reaction and those of several other conditions overlap. Anxiety or fear may cause a quickened pulse, cold hands, and shaking. Too many cups of coffee can produce a nervousness akin to the feelings of a reaction. The hot flashes of menopause or other hormonal changes may mimic hypoglycemia. And a rapidly falling blood sugar level may bring the symptoms of a reaction long before blood sugar really is low. Treating a reaction when your symptoms are actually caused by anxiety may result in a high blood sugar level; so, at first, it is best to test your blood whenever possible to verify that the glucose level really is too low. *However, any time you are in doubt and cannot test, it is much better to eat some rapidly absorbed carbohydrate than risk experiencing a severe reaction.* If the symptoms begin to decrease, it's likely your blood sugar was too low. (Some diabetes educators are finding people with all the symptoms of a reaction whose blood sugar is normal or high. Usually they have had high blood sugar for a long time. If this is the case for you, discuss it with your physician. You should still eat some carbohydrates to relieve your symptoms.)

The symptoms of hypoglycemia can also be masked by the effects of alcohol or other drugs. A person with diabetes who becomes even moderately intoxicated or stoned may not notice a reaction until the blood sugar level is quite low. The need for caution is compounded by alcohol, because this drug lowers blood sugar when one has not eaten for some time. It also blocks the liver's ability to release glucose into the blood. So a couple of drinks before dinner can generate a severe insulin reaction that may not be discovered until the process is already far along. If you do choose to drink or use other drugs, it is best to check your blood sugar level and eat a moderate snack (unless your tests are high—over 180 mg/dl—to begin with).

Somogyi Reactions

One tricky form of insulin reaction has an exotic name, the Somogyi reaction (named for its discoverer, Dr. I. M. Somogyi). This is a prolonged insulin reaction that usually occurs during sleep as the result of too much insulin in the bloodstream. During this special type of reaction, the symptoms usually are not strong enough to wake you; on the other hand, blood sugar does not continue to go down. (Somogyi reactions are different in this way from typical nighttime insulin reactions in which you either wake up in a sweat or don't wake up until the medics pump glucose into your arm.)

The low blood sugar level triggers the body's defense system, and glucose is released along with hormones that attempt to slow down the burning of glucose. A side effect of this process is the burning of fat, resulting in some degree of ketosis (reflected in a positive test for the ketones in the urine). Because of the rebound effect, one may find blood sugar at a relatively high level in the morning and ketones in the urine. If the doctor responds by giving you more insulin, a vicious cycle is started that leads to more and more severe Somogyi reactions. The appropriate response is either a reduction in total insulin dosage or an adjustment in the timing of insulin action.

Signs of a Somogyi reaction:

1. Ketones in the urine, with blood sugar under 250 mg/dl.

2. Evidence of night sweating (wet bedclothes).

3. Low temperature in the morning (body temperature may be low for as long as six hours after an insulin reaction).

4. Bad dreams or nightmares.

5. Grumpiness, abdominal pain, or headache upon awakening.

6. An apparent need for high insulin dosage (more than 50-60 units a day).

If you suspect that you are having Somogyi reactions, discuss your symptoms with your doctor. But first, you should do a bit of research by setting the alarm for a time midway through your sleep period and then testing your blood for several different nights to see if your blood sugar is at hypoglycemic levels (below 60 mg/dl). If so, the component of your insulin dose active during the night will need to be decreased. Usually only a few units are cut, although sometimes the overall insulin dose may be excessive and larger cuts may be needed. (Almost normal bedtime sugars with low or low normal 3:00 A.M. levels and high prebreakfast levels suggest the Somogyi reaction.) *Do not make changes in your basic insulin dosage without talking with your physician.*

A diabetic on the metabolic roller coaster produced by Somogyi reactions is likely to experience strong emotional swings. Such a person may have periods of irritability, depression, or anxiety, together with a sense of fatigue. These feelings are likely to clear when blood sugar levels even out.

Reactions and Optimal Control

In a person who manages diabetes with moderate or loose control, an insulin reaction may represent a very large fall in blood sugar level, and sometimes a very rapid one. The symptoms are usually strong and easily recognized. When stricter control is gained on the intensive regimen, the fall in blood sugar to reaction level may be as little as 20 or 30 mg/dl, and the change may take place very gradually. As a result, the symptoms are often much subtler. Slight confusion or vaguely unclear vision may be the only signs that blood sugar has dipped to 50 or 60 mg/dl. It is clear that those of us who maintain this level of management need to heighten our awareness and not expect all reactions to sound a strong alarm. One of the early findings from the Diabetes Control and Complications Trial (DCCT) is that those on tight control had significantly more severe reactions than those on the looser regimens. Again, the ability to check blood sugar level allows verification of hypoglycemia. In this way, we can learn what our new, subtler set of signals is.

In addition, during the time of switching over to the intensive regimen, reactions are likely to occur more frequently. The cushion against hypoglycemia provided by high blood sugar levels is gone, and it takes time to gain the skills and knowledge necessary to stay in balance. This is one reason for keeping schedules, diet, and exercise as regular as possible during this time. Once you've learned to play the game, you can make changes easily and still stick to the golden mean.

A person with diabetes who is first gaining optimal control may find that even normal blood sugar levels feel rather uncomfortable and trigger symptoms of hypoglycemia. This is especially true if blood sugar levels have been chronically high earlier. This is a brief occurrence, usually lasting no more than a week or two. The symptoms fade after adjustment to a more normal metabolism.

TREATING INSULIN REACTIONS

You now have a choice between making diabetes care a "treat" or a treatment. When blood sugar is too low, the sweets you usually avoid are prescribed medicine. Some of us use this opportunity to satisfy our craving for candy, cookies, and ice cream. Eating these foods is perfectly acceptable as long as you are able to control the amount you eat and not end up bingeing. On the other hand, pharmaceutical companies are now making products designed to treat insulin reactions. These are made of straight glucose—sugar in its most rapidly absorbed form. The advantage of using glucose lies in its somewhat quicker absorption rate, the precisely measured dose, and the fact that glucose products are less likely to lead to overdose or to indiscriminate use when blood sugar is not low. The flavor is rather bland. The disadvantage: They cost more than candy and they're difficult to carry in the pocket.

So long as the sugar is in a form that can be absorbed quickly, the amount used is more important than the kind. The usual recommendation is to eat a food containing 10 to 15 grams of concentrated carbohydrate. Some foods that satisfy this requirements are listed in the accompanying table. For comparison, we also list some dessert servings that would be overkill if taken for a moderate reaction.

Some Appropriate Treats for Insulin Reactions

One-half cup (4 ounces) orange juice — 13 grams carbo

One-half cup apple juice — 15 grams carbo

Six ounces (½ can) cola — 15 grams carbo

One fig bar — 10 grams carbo

Two 2-inch chocolate chip cookies — 12 grams carbo

One tablespoon of granulated sugar — 12 grams carbo

Two teaspoons jam — 14 grams carbo

One-half-ounce raisins (half a small bag) — 10 grams carbo

One-half-ounce caramel or peanut brittle — 12 grams carbo

Five Life Savers — 10 gram carbo

(The wise diabetic carries a couple of servings of these items and keeps a stash in the glove compartment, desk, or locker. A role of Life Savers is especially convenient and inconspicuous.)

Some Excessive Treats

One slice apple pie — 60 grams carbo (four times as much as you need)

One piece of cake with frosting — 60 grams carbo

Twelve ounces of cola (a full can or bottle) — 30 grams carbo (twice times the necessary amount)

One jelly doughnut — 48 grams carbo (three times as much as you need)

When you are in the throes of a full-tilt insulin reaction—confused, pulse racing, anxious, and extremely hungry—the temptation to overdose is powerful, to say the least. (This is especially true in the middle of the night, when blood sugar may fall to a very low level before you wake up.) If you wish to avoid an enormous leap in blood sugar level, however, you are advised to learn to eat moderately. Treat reactions in stages, first eating a sweet in the category of 10 to 15 grams of carbohydrate, waiting ten or fifteen minutes, and then taking another sweet only if the symptoms have not disappeared. (The obvious exception to this practice would be when you are experiencing a very severe reaction following heavy exercise or a missed meal. At such a time, you may need to double the amount of sugar to bring blood glucose back to normal.) Remember that you are likely to have a rebound effect, with the glucose from your liver increasing blood sugar, along with the sugar you use to treat the reaction. If you overeat, your next blood test may be up in the 300s.

Unless the reaction occurs within an hour of mealtime, you should have a moderate snack of longer-acting food—whole grain bread, crackers and cheese, nuts—after you have eaten a sweet. This will tide you over to the next meal and prevent another reaction.

As an insulin-dependent diabetic, you run the risk of not waking up when a reaction occurs, or of becoming unconscious because hypoglycemia is not treated in time. The people close to you should know what to do if they find you unconscious, so ask them to read this next section and take notes.

To the Person Who May Need to Treat an Unconscious Diabetic . . .

If you find that you cannot rouse your sleeping beauty, it is most likely that he or she is in insulin shock (severe hypoglycemia or insulin reaction), the result of very low blood sugar. The accompanying table compares the outward symptoms of insulin shock and diabetic coma (the result of very high blood sugar), so you can know for sure what is happening.

If it looks as if your friend is in a diabetic coma, the only treatment you can institute is calling a physician and getting him or her into the hospital immediately. If the doctor is not available, get your friend to an emergency room. Probably he or she will not have been feeling well for the last half-day or more. Diabetic coma is gradual in onset, and usually one feels ill, is thirsty, and has to urinate frequently as the process unfolds.

Outward Signs of Insulin Shock and Diabetic Coma

Shock	Coma
Sudden onset (minutes to hours)	Gradual onset (days)
Pale, moist, sweaty skin	Flushed, dry skin
Shallow breathing	Deep, labored breathing
Normal breath	Fruity smell on breath
Rapid pulse	Usually rapid pulse
Low blood sugar	Very high blood sugar

If the patient is in insulin shock, you may be able to help him or her regain consciousness on your own. Provide sugar in a form that he or she won't choke on. The best possible treatment is glucagon, a substance injected just like insulin. If you're lucky, there is a kit around and you have been instructed in its use. There are two vials— one containing the dry glucagon and the other, sterile water. You mix the two with the syringe and inject the mixture under the skin in a fleshy spot like the thigh or back of the arm. The glucagon encourages the liver to release glucose.

If there is no glucagon, jam or jelly is the treatment of choice, or a tube of frosting, or one of the jellied glucose products like Glutose or Monojel. Rub a bit on your friend's lips and into the mouth with your fingers, and he or she may start sucking. Stroke the throat to encourage swallowing. Provide a couple of tablespoons or more. (Ernest's wife, Grace, revived him once with an appropriately named preserve—Hero's Jam.)

If nothing is available in jellied form, see if you can get your friend to swallow very small sips of any fruit juice or soda pop (not diet soda!). Be cautious—you don't want to cause choking. Don't try any solid sweet unless you can get enough response to be sure that it will be chewed and swallowed and not cause gagging.

The scarcity of blood sugar reaching the diabetic's brain may produce antagonism and uncooperativeness as he or she starts to revive. It may seem like poor thanks for all you've just been through, but don't be alarmed. It's a natural result of a serious insulin reaction.

If you're not sure whether it's diabetic coma or insulin shock, it's best to try giving a sweet (as above) to see what happens. Low blood sugar can cause harm more quickly than high blood sugar.

If your patient doesn't start to recover consciousness within five minutes by the clock, call the medic team or get him or her to an emergency room. You've done everything you can. Thank you for your loving care.

To the Person with Diabetes . . .

Show your love for the people close to you by not putting them through the process just described. It is one of the most terrifying events that can be inflicted on someone. Study the next section on preventing reactions carefully, and practice what you learn here. If you have had more than one reaction that you did not awaken from in recent years, we suggest that you do the exercise on page 183.

PREVENTING INSULIN REACTIONS

The most fundamental way to avoid reactions is to be willing to keep a corner of your awareness devoted to diabetes. Don't obsess about it, but simply acknowledge that it is a companion who refuses to be left behind. People who suffer from frequent insulin reactions are often the ones who try to pretend that they do not have diabetes. This clearly doesn't work, and they often end up with vivid reminders of their illness.

You are more likely to have an insulin reaction in certain situations. When you have been more active, when a meal is delayed, or when you have eaten lightly, it is easy to predict that hypoglycemia will occur if you don't compensate for the change in routine. If these situations become cues to awareness, like little alarm clocks, you will find that you automatically take the appropriate action. The light meal or the delay becomes a signal for an added snack (unless blood sugar tests are high).

To deal with an increase in activity level, you can either take less insulin (cutting dose by two or three units, up to one-third the total dose, depending on the amount of the increase in exercise), or you can increase your food intake. A good rule of thumb is to eat 10 to 15 grams additional carbohydrate for each thirty minutes of extra physical activity (a slice of bread, a whole double graham cracker, one-half-ounce of raisins, or a medium orange).

Through trial and error you will find the amount that's right for the kind of activities you are involved in. You will be able to hike or work all afternoon in the garden and keep in balance, avoiding both reactions and high blood sugar. The chart of calorie expenditures in Chapter 10, "Living Actively With Diabetes," gives you an idea of how much food you burn up with different activities. Note that vigorous activities (digging with a shovel, playing tennis, or hiking uphill) can use close to a whole meal's worth of calories in one hour.

Remember that vigorous exercise continues to lower blood sugar for as much as four to six hours after you finish; you may need an extra snack or a larger meal after a period of prolonged or intense activity. This happens because well-exercised muscles absorb more sugar from the bloodstream, even after the activity stops. Exercising regularly in itself helps you avoid reactions; the glucose stored in the muscles can be drawn on when the blood sugar level goes down.

Diet is another factor that helps to stabilize blood sugar levels and prevent hypoglycemia. If you tend to eat the slower-burning foods, you will have a more continuous supply of glucose entering the blood-stream. This is one reason the high complex carbohydrate, high fiber diet is being recommended by many nutritionists. Protein burns even slower, but it is usually accompanied by more fat than we need.

As you become more aware of the physical sensations that precede an insulin reaction, you will find that you can often eat just enough simple carbohydrate to stay at a normal blood sugar level and neither fall into hypoglycemia nor jump up to a high level. You gain a sense of "dosage" with foods like raisins, prunes, and fresh fruit. ("There's that feeling. I could test, but there's no reason to think that I have anything but normal or low blood sugar. Let's see, four prunes should see me through to lunch.") Sometimes this becomes a matter of shifting the order of a meal, eating the fruit or other simple carbohydrate at the beginning of the meal rather than at the end. Anyone who has experienced the frustration of a reaction occurring while gulping down a meal that won't be absorbed for an hour knows the value of this practice.

Developing an Early Warning System

Sensitivity to the symptoms of insulin reactions varies greatly from person to person. One may be very aware of bodily states, noting the beginning of hypoglycemia at a very early stage. Another may be so absorbed in day-to-day activities that he or she recognizes a reaction only when sweat is already pouring down the brow and speech is slurred. You can take steps to increase your bodily awareness and thereby your chances for survival. Diabetic neuropathy (see Chapter 17) and certain prescription drugs (such as beta blockers prescribed for high blood pressure or heart disease) can also block the typical symptoms. "Hypoglycemic unawareness" from less clear causes is also becoming more widely observed.

Also, a few diabetics have rare hormone deficiencies that mask or even eliminate the symptoms of hypoglycemia. Blood sugar may fall to very low levels before any symptoms are experienced. Unfortunately, the symptoms that do occur are likely to be confusion or emotional instability caused by the brain receiving too little glucose. Frequent blood testing and meticulous adherence to regimen is especially important for anyone in this category.

Many of us can sense the approach of an insulin reaction before blood sugar reaches a hypoglycemic level. It is possible to cultivate sensitivity to the subtle cues your body gives that indicate you are about to bottom out. This calls for deepening physical awareness, something that many diabetics avoid. When blood sugar is chronically high (200+ mg/dl), we tend to be mildly uncomfortable. (Ernest describes his discomfort as the feeling of having fine sand or granules of sugar in his muscles.) Rather than experience this vague distress, many of us ignore our bodies and live in our heads. Reactions have to be thundering before we notice them. If you spend much time out of touch with your body, there are ways you can increase your bodily awareness.

One way is to make routine physical activities like brushing your teeth, shaving, or showering occasions for *feeling* your body rather than thinking about other things. Become aware, for instance, of the sensation of temperature in various body parts, muscle tensions, the texture of whatever surface is in contact with your skin, the feeling of your breath or pulse. (When you are relatively quiet you can sense the pulsing of your whole circulatory system.) A particularly good time for this casual survey is when you have time available because you are waiting for something to happen. Your body is always happening—no waiting necessary!

A more direct way of heightening physical awareness is to focus closely on everything you experience in your body as you become hypoglycemic (and, of course, as you eat something). See how many different sensations you can notice. Make mental notes. See how the sensations may differ from time to time. (More techniques are described in Chapter 11, "Living Well With Stress.")

Along with generally increasing body awareness, you can use blood testing to help identify the early cues that a reaction is near. When you note a physical change that might be signaling the approach of low blood sugar, check to see what your level actually is. If you are still in the normal range (70-120) wait a few minutes and see if more distinct reaction symptoms develop. (A reaction is more likely to follow a normal blood sugar reading of 80 than a reading of 120.) If you do this occasionally and write down the cues that are followed by a reaction, you will soon find that you can act to bring blood sugar level up before the stronger symptoms have developed. A real advantage here is that you avoid the rebound to high blood sugar levels produced by the stress of a full-scale reaction.

If you have difficulty waking up at night when blood sugar plummets, there are two solutions, one mental and one medical. The first is a matter of suggesting to yourself that you are ready and willing to learn to pay attention to the alarm your body rings, no matter what time it sounds. This can be done as a gentle talk with your body while you are relaxing into sleep, a time when your mind is very open to suggestion. You can find your own words to express thoughts such as these: "Body, I know that you send me signals when a reaction is happening and I want you to know that I am willing to hear them, no matter how deeply I am sleeping. I don't want to put you through the stress that occurs when I fail to wake up. I want to live well with you and our special needs. I'm willing to hear your call for help." You can reinforce the message by remembering the sensations that usually tell you a reaction is beginning and seeing an image of yourself awakening, getting out of bed, and going to the kitchen for a 3:00 A.M. snack. You can also use this sort of process to reinforce your awareness of daytime hypoglycemia.

The mechanical solution to not waking up when reactions occur is based on the wet bedclothes that we have all discovered in the middle of the night. The sweat of a strong reaction triggers a mechanical moisture sensor under the bedding that sets off an alarm. There is also a sweat sensor called The Sleep Sentry that can be worn on the wrist. (Ask your pharmacist or the diabetic supply firms listed in the Appendix about these products.)

As we mentioned earlier, certain types of stress can have a hypoglycemic effect. Relatively little is known about stress and diabetes, but it may be true that active expression of emotion, especially strong anger, tends to lower blood sugar. (The opposite—silent stewing and depression—appear to raise blood sugar.) What we can say with certainty is that you should study the effects on you of different kinds of stress so you will now which ones might cause insulin reactions. Then you will know when you may need to take preventive steps.

With a Little Help. . .

There is a social side to preventing insulin reactions. People close to you and those with whom you work have a right to know that you have diabetes and what the outward signs of hypoglycemia are for you. It is unwise to risk a situation dangerous for you and difficult for others because of pride. There are times when one is concentrating strongly on an activity or when confusion is the first symptom to appear. At such times, someone else may notice the signs of hypoglycemia long before you do. Make it easy for anyone to ask if you are having a reaction if they think this might be happening.

Another social aspect of reactions is that some of us feel embarrassed and a bother to others when we need food fast, especially if this interrupts or changes planned activities. It can be difficult to say, "I can't wait until we get to the beach to eat. Can we stop now? I have a reaction." But you will be putting your friends to much greater bother if you pass out on them while trying to remain "inconspicuous." You will find that if you state your needs directly, most people will be understanding. A variation on this pattern of embarrassment is feeling self-conscious about eating in front of others who are not eating, especially when they think of you as someone who "shouldn't" eat sweets.

If you are about to engage in a public performance, such as giving a talk or making a long sales call, you may feel anxious about the possibility of becoming hypoglycemic. The anxiety may even feel like a reaction. If possible, test your blood sugar beforehand and eat enough to get you through if it is not already high. If you can't test, go ahead and have a moderate snack. The risk of one high test is certainly less than the risk of falling apart at an important moment. (The precaution here is doubly important when the performance involves physical activity.)

We hope that the practice of wearing a diabetes I.D. bracelet or necklace and carrying a card with details of insulin dosage can be taken for granted. Unfortunately, some of us are afraid to have our friends or co-workers identify us with diabetes, and neglect to wear this basic bit of jewelry. In an episode of insulin shock or an accident, it could save your life.

SOME QUESTIONABLE BENEFITS OF REACTIONS

If you seem to resist doing anything to reduce the number of reactions you have, you may be gaining hidden benefits from them. The simplest example of this: When you are hypoglycemic, it is medically prescribed to eat something you are normally discouraged from eating ("Oh boy, a sweet treat! This is a pretty strong one. I must need a hot fudge sundae or apple pie a la mode"). Children are not the only ones to cultivate reactions as an excuse to indulge. As we mentioned before, when the sugar of the food joins with the rebound effect, you are likely to end up with a blood sugar level much higher than if you had eaten the candy without having a reaction.

The solution is also simple: Don't use the reaction to gain something you can just go ahead and do. In this case, give yourself a vacation once in a while and eat something sweet. It will help if you do it when your blood sugar level is near normal or when you are planning to be more active than usual. If you're going to be really outrageous (hot fudge sundae level), you might take an extra unit or two of rapid-acting insulin just before you gorge (but not at bedtime!). So long as this doesn't happen too often or lead to a binge, your control will be much steadier than if you go on having reactions in order to eat sweets. It is best not to use a big dessert as a substitute for a meal. It's possible you'll end up with a major reaction because the concentrated carbo-hydrate is absorbed rapidly and you have no continuing source of glucose.

Some of us use hypoglycemia as permission to express hostility we normally keep bottled up. Some of the sweetest diabetics rant and rage when their blood sugar level falls too low. Anyone who suggests that they may need a few chocolate chip cookies becomes a target for their abuse. When it is all over, the insulin reaction, not the person is held responsible. If this is your pattern, the direct approach to living is the key to living well. Learn to express your anger directly.

There are other ways some people with diabetes use reactions to escape responsibility. Not waking up from a reaction at night is practically a guaranteed method of getting someone else to take care of you. When you are knocked out by hypoglycemia, someone else has to play Mother to bring you out of it. It can become a way of testing a mate or a parent: "If you really love me, you'll save my life." It can also be a form of revenge, given the amount of stress the rescuer must go through to revive you. Ironically, the diabetic who fails to wake up at night may be the very one who fights off all assistance when he or she is hypoglycemic during the day, saying, "Don't you think I can take care of myself?"

An Anecdote

Two couples in one of the support groups Ernest ran in California played identical games around reactions. Each of the two men had experienced repeated nighttime hypoglycemia that had to be treated by their wives or the medic team. The men insisted they couldn't do anything about it. The wives were growing increasingly frustrated and angry.

When reactions occurred during the day, the men insisted on their independence and ability to take care of themselves. They were very reluctant to pay attention to the reaction cues their wives would point out in the evening, often waiting until they were deep into hypoglycemia to eat something. It took the feedback of the whole support group to help the men see the pattern of dependence they were caught in. They and their wives had to work to form a more balanced relationship.

This is a delicate issue to work with. We want to be independent, yet we must depend on food as well as insulin. We depend on regularity of meals. We depend on doctors to help us handle our condition and its complications. And, worst of all, in a very fundamental way, we cannot depend on our own bodies as others do. No wonder we sometimes bounce back and forth between declaring our independence and acting very dependent.

If you suspect that a desire to be taken care of is at the root of your difficulties with insulin reactions, you might explore the question with those who are important to you. In what ways can you be more direct in asking for care and support? What can you give in return? And, most important, what can you give yourself to increase your sense of being well cared for?

REACTIONS AND SEX

One of the peak frustrations in a diabetic's life occurs when the passion drains away just before or while making love, and an insulin reaction takes the place of an orgasm. The wisdom of the body makes the wise choice of preservation over reproduction and pleasure; but sometimes that's not easy to explain to your partner. So this is one more time when a pre-event blood test and a little extra food may be in order, especially if you tend to be an athletic lover.

187

Section III
LIVING WELL WITH THE KEYS TO CONTROL

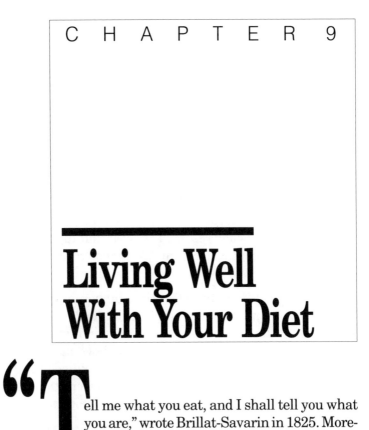

C H A P T E R 9

Living Well With Your Diet

"Tell me what you eat, and I shall tell you what you are," wrote Brillat-Savarin in 1825. Moreover, food and eating are an inextricable part of our culture, from daily activities (the coffee break) to major events (the Thanksgiving feast). Edward Espe Brown, a Zen priest, fine poet, great chef, and cookbook writer, wrote in 1991 that "food is not just food, something 'out there'; food is our body, the body of the world, the way the body of the world becomes our body . . . . Eating with awareness, we know that life is delicious . . . . We join again the ageless dance of life—and rejoice." These words are especially meaningful to people with diabetes. Food and eating are very important parts of our lives. Most of us are very conscious of how particular foods, the quantities we eat, and when we eat them, affect how we feel. Nutritional research has radically revised our understanding of the effects of various foods on our metabolism.

In this chapter, we highlight how the recommended "diabetic diet" has changed over the years, describe new findings, and integrate these into guidelines for healthy, appealing meals. We will also share some

191

personal tips on ways to enjoy food and eating within these guidelines. In the process, we will watch old nutritional dogma become myth.

THE SO-CALLED DIABETIC DIET

Before insulin was discovered, people with diabetes were instructed to completely avoid carbohydrates (starches and sugars). After insulin was discovered, those with diabetes were usually put on low-carbohydrate diets with moderately high fat and protein. (Paradoxically, in the 1920s and 1930s, some research showed that high-carbohydrate diets may be more advantageous than low-carbohydrate ones, but this work was largely ignored.)

The exchange system, based on the number of grams (weight) of the carbohydrate, protein, and fat in each food, became the basis for determining the proper diet for an individual with diabetes. Usually the patient's physician would decide how many calories seemed appropriate, refer the patient to a dietitian skilled in teaching patients about exchange groups, create a diet prescription, tailor it to the patient's preferences, and issue warnings about which foods to avoid.

By the 1960s and 1970s, many physicians were recommending diets that were more flexible and less rigid, basing this recommendation mainly on the experiences of their patients. Little new research was being done, and different doctors perpetuated different truths—and myths—to their patients. However, by the mid-seventies, Americans were becoming more food conscious, and the effects of various foods on health were becoming more widely known. Along with growing interest in nutrition, sophisticated research was adding new and better data, which were widely disseminated to the general public.

Recommendations included decreasing the cholesterol, total fat, and saturated animal or vegetable fats in our diets, increasing the proportion of unsaturated fats and mono-unsaturated fats (like olive oil) to saturated fats, and increasing the amount of fruit, vegetables, and fiber in our daily meals. Not surprisingly, these guidelines are totally appropriate for diabetics.

What was new and especially important for diabetics was research on effect of specific foods on blood sugar levels in healthy people. This research turned up some surprising findings. Certain foods that diabetics had always been told to avoid, like ice cream, raised the blood sugar only half as much as "good" foods like whole wheat bread. Nutritionists were finding that the glycemic effect (impact on blood sugar level) of a particular food was determined by a variety of factors, not simply by the number of grams of carbohydrate. The physical form of the food and the amount of fat eaten with it seemed to make a major difference in the food's effects.

Before we look at these recommendations in more detail, you might want to answer the following questions.

1. Among the foods you eat regularly, which do you enjoy the most? _____

_____

2. Which of the above foods, if any, do you consider healthy? Which do you consider unhealthy?_____

_____

3. What foods would you like to eat more of, but don't, because you feel they are unhealthy?_____

_____

4. What foods do you eat too much of?_____

_____

Review your answers to these questions. You may change some of your judgments about "good" and "bad" foods as you learn new information in this chapter.

NEW FACTS ABOUT FOOD

Fat and Cholesterol

Most scientists and health professionals now agree that we all would be better off if we decreased the total fat in our diets, increased the ratio of polyunsaturated and mono-unsaturated fats to saturated fats, and reduced our cholesterol intake. Total fat, and especially saturated fat, in our diet is the major factor affecting our cholesterol levels, even more than the amount of cholesterol we eat. (Polyunsaturated fats include most liquid vegetable oils; a major mono-unsaturated fat is olive oil; saturated fats are all animal fats, including dairy fats, and coconut and palm oil.) These changes have been linked to reduced risk of heart disease in nondiabetics. Since people with diabetes have twice the risk of heart disease as the general population, these dietary guidelines are especially important.

The American Diabetes Association, as well as the British and Canadian diabetes associations, have recommended lowering the fat content of diabetic diets from the usual 40 to 45 percent of total calories to less than 30 percent. The gap needs to be filled with more calories from either carbohydrate ("carbo") or protein. Recent studies generally have shown no serious adverse effects from high-carbo diets, especially when most of the calories come from complex carbohydrates (starches) with associated fiber. The ADA recommends 50 to 60 percent of calories from carbohydrates, minimizing simple sugars. (That leaves 15 to 20 percent from protein.) More about carbos later when we discuss the glycemic index.

What about cholesterol? Doctors are increasingly recommending moderate intake of cholesterol. A large-scale study called "The Lipid Research Clinics Coronary Primary Prevention Trial" looked at middle-aged men who had no evidence of heart disease but did have cholesterol levels of 265 mg/dl or higher. This study showed that diet and the drug cholestyramine not only lowered cholesterol levels, but also reduced the risk of heart attack. This research provided strong evidence, for the first time, that decreasing cholesterol may directly prevent the development of coronary heart disease.

This report and a growing body of other evidence prompted the National Institutes of Health to convene a conference with a panel of fourteen experts to examine cholesterol and heart disease. This panel made the following recommendations:

1. All Americans over age 2 should adopt a diet limiting total fat to 30 percent (just as in the American Diabetes Association's plan). No more than one-third of the fat should be saturated,

and cholesterol should be limited to 250-300 mg a day. (A large egg yolk, a very concentrated form of cholesterol, has almost that much.)

2. Target levels for normal values among adults should be: under 30 years old, blood cholesterol no higher that 180 mg/dl; over 30, blood cholesterol no higher than 200 mg/dl. (These levels are below what many physicians consider acceptable, and are probably below the actual average levels for Americans.)

Most of you know that total cholesterol is made up of the "good" HDL cholesterol and the "bad" cholesterols, LDL and VLDL. Many experts feel that it is important to know your HDL level, especially if your total cholesterol is high. They believe that the ratio of total cholesterol to HDL cholesterol is the most significant number for determining risk. For example, if your total cholesterol is 200 and your HDL is 50, your ratio is 200÷50=4, which is good. (Any ratio under 4.5 is considered good.)

What does this mean for us? That it has become increasingly easy for people with diabetes to eat low-fat, low-cholesterol diets. More attention has been given to labels on foods. Manufacturers and restaurants are offering more low-fat and fat-free products. There is more support for these practices among the general population. The "diabetic diet" is good for everyone.

There have been several news items recently casting doubt on the benefits of "healthy eating." However, we believe that for people with diabetes, the benefits far outweigh the "costs." For example, some of you may have heard about the "French paradox," where the French apparently eat much more fat than we do, yet have a much lower rate of heart disease. Or you may have read about the study that calculated that the average American would live only three to four months longer by following a 30 percent fat diet. Well, it seems that years ago the French had a diet much lower in fat than currently, and that the heart disease rate is likely to rise as those with the current diet age. And the mathematical study averaged the benefits over all individuals, not only those who might benefit the most. Probably researchers will find that some of us have genes that will protect us no matter what we eat. However, today we know that those with diabetes are already at high risk for heart disease, and the odds are that following a low-fat diet will benefit us.

Fiber

Food scientists and health professionals have increasing evidence that dietary fiber is good for those with diabetes. High fiber intake lowers cholesterol levels, lowers the usual rise in blood sugar following meals, and decreases insulin requirements.

The fiber we are talking about is plant fiber, the kind found in vegetables, fruits, grains, and legumes (beans). It is useful to divide fiber into two types: soluble (guar and pectin) and insoluble. The soluble is found in fruits, dried beans, and oat products (or in a pure form extracted from them); insoluble fiber is in other grains, wheat (cereal) bran, and vegetables. Soluble fiber lowers cholesterol.

How does fiber work? In general, the water-soluble fibers slow down the time food, particularly glucose, takes to leave the stomach, pass through the intestine, and be absorbed into the bloodstream. Soluble fiber increases the viscosity (thickness) of food in the digestive tract. On the other hand, insoluble fibers act like roughage and increase the bulk of our stool. Soluble fiber has a more acute effect on our blood sugar, smoothing out the response to food, whereas the insoluble fiber has a more long-term effect (two to three weeks) on glucose tolerance. Thus, it's wise to eat both kinds of fiber.

We can increase our fiber intake simply by eating more fresh fruits and vegetables, beans, bran, and whole grain. (See Table 2 at the end of this chapter.) Many health-food products are available to add purified fiber to the diet, but these must be mixed into the food in order to affect the glycemic response. We favor the fiber found in natural plant sources rather than these supplements.

The Glycemic Effect

Traditionally, carbohydrates have been divided into simple and complex groups. Simple carbos consist of refined sugar and the unprocessed sugar found in fruits and vegetables; complex carbos consist of starches found in potatoes, rice, other grains, and beans. People with diabetes have been taught to avoid simple sugars, in the belief that they were absorbed more quickly and raised the blood sugar higher and faster than starches. Recent research has shown that the biologic effect of food on blood sugar is much more complex. It is clear, however, that proteins and fats will not raise blood sugar substantially, unless eaten in large amounts.

Under test conditions, researchers have found that some foods earlier thought to have less rapid effects on blood sugar (like potatoes) raise blood sugar as rapidly as a Mars bar. And other foods, like ice cream, raise blood sugar half as fast as a starchy staple like bread. Various foods have been studied and compared to the effect of pure glucose on blood sugar. Glucose was assigned a glycemic index of 100, and all other foods received a score proportional to the pure glucose effect. More recently, the standard has been changed so that one slice of white bread equals 100, and the scores adjusted appropriately (see Table 1 at the end of this chapter). Foods with a low glycemic index are called slow releasers.

What have these studies taught us? First, that pure sugars are high, but table sugar (sucrose) is less than bread (only 86), and fructose a low 30. (You still need to limit them, however, because of their high concentration.) High-fat foods, like ice cream and pastry, have relatively low indices, whether they are simple or complex carbos. (Fat is thought to slow absorption of carbohydrates.) Grain products vary widely, but there is little difference between whole grain and white bread, or whole grain and white pasta (spaghetti, noodles, etc.) The difference between pasta and bread is considerable. Pasta is a very slow releaser, thus raising blood sugar level much less than most other grain products.

The physical form of the food appears to explain the differences between pasta and bread. The starch in the pasta is more compact and perhaps less accessible to digestive enzymes. Similarly, rice ground into flour results in higher glycemic levels than does rice as a whole grain. Legumes (beans and peas), as a food group, have the lowest index. Presumably, their soluble fiber increases food viscosity, slows movement through the gut, and slows absorption. Finally, most cooked root vegetables, like white potatoes, beets, and carrots, have a very high index as a group. However, an average serving of cooked carrots has only 5 grams of carbo. Surprisingly, sweet potatoes and yams (not candied) have relatively low glycemic indices.

A few words of caution here: Although a food like ice cream has a low glycemic index, it should not be eaten in large quantities or substituted for potatoes. The fat and cholesterol in ice cream must also be considered. Also, the high candy content of some flavors (like English toffee or raspberry jamocha fudge ripple) should be considered nearly the same as straight candy.

An interesting observation we have made, and confirmed with others (although we have seen no published studies), is the high glycemic effect of Indian and Chinese food. This is independent of the obvious sources of carbo like rice or flour products.

Researchers are still disagreeing on how this new information should be applied. Nevertheless, we believe that we can offer reasonable guidelines on the basis of experience. Suggestions on how best to use the glycemic index are incorporated into the recommendations in the next section.

NUTRITION GUIDELINES

These guidelines are based on the preceding information, current ADA recommendations, and our own and others' experiences. Under each guideline, we will add tips that make the recommendation easier to follow.

Work with your physician or a dietitian to establish a general plan for total calories, distributed as mentioned earlier among carbos, mono-unsaturated, polyunsaturated, and saturated fat, protein (and alcohol, if desired). One gram of carbo or protein equals 4 calories, one gram of fat equals 9 calories, and one gram of alcohol about 7 calories. The calorie conversion will greatly assist you in reading labels and calculating the percentage of calories from fat and the other food groups. For example, if the label says one serving is 150 calories and that the amount of fat is 10 grams, multiply the number of grams of fat (10) by 9 calories, equaling 90 calories of the 150 from fat (60% of calories from fat).

Use Moderation

This principle is a guiding rule that will almost always keep you out of trouble. What you eat typically, frequently, or habitually (e.g. every day for breakfast, 3 days a week at work, every night while watching television) is what will have the most impact. What you eat every once in a while is far less important.

1. Become a taster. Eat just a bite or two of a food that would greatly raise your blood sugar if you ate the whole thing.

2. Even slowly absorbed foods such as pasta should be eaten in the proper amounts. Too large a serving will produce high blood sugar tests later in the day. Be moderate also with high-fat foods, such as nuts and nut butters or potato chips. An ounce of peanuts has 165 calories, even more when cooked in oil.

3. Share sweet desserts with friends when you want a treat. Satisfy your craving without overloading your system. (You may have to explain to people that small servings of dessert are not poison to a diabetic.)

4. You may fear that sugar lust will overcome you, and one bite will lead to a binge. Since binges are usually a secret activity, you can learn to control this urge by eating sweets only when you are with other people. Say, "I'm going to eat three bits of this pie and then it's all yours."

Ernie and the Microchips

> *I managed to acquire a taste for Swiss chocolate in the last few years, in spite of its high fat content. Bittersweet, especially, doesn't have that much sugar, I told myself. And traditionally I'd worried more about sugar than fats. Then I decided to break with tradition and cut my dietary fat content fairly drastically. Give up chocolate? Well, how about less? And I find the flavor is so intense that I can now thoroughly enjoy eating two or three microchips— a half inch square weighing a few grams—where before I would have eaten a whole section of a bar. Principle: moderation enables us to enjoy.*

Decrease Total Fat, Saturated Fat, and Cholesterol

1. Eat less red meat. When you do eat it, choose cuts that have little fat. Limit your consumption of fast-food hamburgers. McDonald's new McLean Deluxe Burger has half the fat of the Quarter Pounder (only 28% of calories from fat) and tastes pretty good. Other fast food chains are also offering low-fat items. Most will provide you with nutritional analysis of their foods upon request. *Fast Food Facts* is a very useful compendium of nutritional values for fast food restaurants (see references at end of chapter).

2. Eat more poultry, but don't eat the skin and fat (except for a small taste). You can broil or grill chicken with the skin removed if you baste it with vegetable oil or an oily marinade.

3. Substitute turkey or chicken products for fatty beef and pork, hot dogs, bologna, and ground meats. But don't always assume that the poultry alternative is lower in fat—do the calculations. Also, try Morningstar Farm products, made from soy. It may take some time to get accustomed to these soy products, but they are worth the effort. Taste preferences are surprisingly changeable.

4. Use low-fat or nondairy products. Certain cheeses, like hoop or farmer cheese and skim milk mozzarella, are lower in fat than others. Fat-free sour cream and lower fat cream cheese are now widely available and almost indistinguishable from the high-fat products.

5. Substitute fish, bean, or tofu for fatty red meat. Fish oil, contained in all fish, is the most unsaturated oil you can eat (about twice as beneficial as vegetable oils).

A word of advice here: Don't take fish oil capsules. They are expensive, they offer no obvious benefit, and they may be harmful. Eat fatty cold-water fish like salmon, trout, haddock, and mackerel instead. They also contain the largest quantity of fats, known as omega-3 fatty acids, that help lower cholesterol and triglycerides and prevent blood clots by thinning the blood.

Furthermore, most seafood is now thought to be relatively low in cholesterol. Although researchers now believe that what was thought to be cholesterol also includes similar appearing fish sterols, it is still unclear just how much cholesterol is in shellfish like shrimp, lobster, and crab. But because they are low in saturated fats, most researchers now believe these are fine to eat in moderation. Mollusks, like scallops, clams, and oysters, are even lower in cholesterol.

Tofu is rapidly becoming a staple of delicious, healthy cooking. This soybean product is itself quite bland, so you can bestow many different flavors on it by your choice of recipes. With the water pressed out, tofu can be grilled (prepared in your favorite marinade first) or crumbled, sautéed, and substituted for ground beef in Mexican and Italian recipes. It is high in protein and contains no cholesterol, but gets about 50 percent of its calories from fat.

The fat in ground meat can be greatly reduced by crumbling it up, simmering it in water, some wine, and some garlic powder and cumin for about fifteen minutes, then draining. The meat can then be used in other recipes or frozen for later use (see references for *Health Smart Gourmet Cooking* at end of chapter). Very low fat ground beef is also available in the meat or frozen sections of your supermarket. Sometimes the fat is replaced by water bound to a food product like carrageenan, a naturally occurring carbohydrate extracted from seaweed.

6. Eat egg yolks and organ meats (liver, kidneys, sweetbreads, etc.) no more than once a week. These are extremely high in cholesterol. The yolk of the egg contains all the cholesterol. You can safely eat egg whites, which are all protein.

7. Use margarine instead of butter. Choose a diet or imitation margarine—one that lists liquid vegetable oil as the first ingredient. (Ingredients are listed on product labels in order of amount, with the highest listed first. Liquid is better than partially hydrogenated oil.) If you prefer to use butter on some foods, use whipped butter in moderate amounts, or mix butter and margarine together.

8. Use noncaloric sprays (Pam and others) when you sauté or fry foods. The good browned flavor that fat adds to sauces can be duplicated by repeated pan reductions of vegetables, sautéed and deglazed with broth or wine. You might want to start with 1-2 teaspoons of vegetable oil.

9. Try Butter Buds, Best O' Butter, or similar products (available in your grocery store), sprinkled on dry or dissolved in water, for adding a buttery flavor to vegetables or popcorn. They have no fat or cholesterol. Low-fat (or nonfat) buttermilk adds wonderful buttery-rich flavor to sauces and mashed potatoes.

10. Use olive oil in salad dressings and for sautéing. Nutritionists once considered mono-unsaturated fats like olive oil to be "neutral" compared to polyunsaturated (good) and saturated fats (bad). Newer research has determined that olive oil is a good fat, particularly in terms of lowering the bad cholesterol (LDL) and raising the good cholesterol (HDL).

11. Eat less total fat. The total fat you eat—particularly saturated fat—is the major dietary factor in determining your cholesterol level. An easy way to estimate the maximum amount of fat to eat each day is to divide your optimum weight in half. Saturated fat should be less than one-third of that (e.g., if your optimum weight for your height is 150 lbs., you should eat no more than 75 grams total fat and 25 grams saturated fat). Remember, even if one particular food has a high percentage of its calories from fat, it can be offset by a low percentage fat food. It's the *daily* total of calories from fat that counts.

12. Limit your intake of saturated vegetable fats like palm and coconut oil. These are used in preparing canned nuts, cheap cookies and candy, and other processed foots. Many manufacturers are eliminating them in response to public opinion. Check the labels.

13. Be on the lookout for a wide variety of low-fat, low-calorie frozen meals or meals "in-a-cup." Also look for low-calorie, low-fat frozen desserts (Weight Watchers makes several varieties). Be sure to do the percentage of fat calculations, and confirm the

amount of carbohydrate (sometimes the carbohydrate remains very high even in foods sweetened with NutraSweet). You can also check the effects of these "new" foods on your blood sugar levels by testing one to two hours after eating.

14. Now available on your grocery shelves are a selection of nonfat salad dressings, mayonnaise, and cheeses! Some taste great, others are OK. The cheeses are particularly good for adding texture or consistency in cooking or for melting onto chili, etc. The fat replacers tend to be either carbo or protein based, so again be sure to check the amounts to determine how they should fit into your eating plan.

Eat Foods with High Fiber and Low Glycemic Index

Don't eliminate foods solely because of their high glycemic index, but do shift the balance. Eat pasta, beans, and fresh fruit more often than potatoes, rice, and bread.

As you increase the carbo in your diet, it is important also to increase the fiber to gain the full beneficial effect: High fiber may be more beneficial when eaten in a high-carbo diet (see Table 2 at the end of this chapter).

Finally, using the tool of home blood glucose testing, you can determine you own glycemic responses to various foods by measuring your blood glucose one or two hours after eating. Let your home tests and blood lipid (fat) levels, as determined by your physician, be your guide in balancing your diet.

Here are some ideas on using fiber and the glycemic index in your diet:

1. Begin to eat more pasta and beans in all their various forms. Choose a slow-release over a fast-release carbo.

2. Eat more fresh fruits and cut down on fruit juices, particularly frozen ones.

3. Popcorn is a wonderful high-fiber, low-calorie food, especially without butter or margarine. To season it, use herbs or spices instead of salt.

4. Look for packaged or processed foods that use fructose instead of sugar or corn syrup. Fructose has a lower glycemic effect.

5. Use nonnutritive sweeteners and products that contain them. Aspartame (NutraSweet or Equal) is now widely available. Use the powdered form very lightly instead of powdered sugar on berries or pancakes, for instance. But use it sparingly, as it's highly concentrated. *Do not cook with Equal. It deteriorates when heated to boiling.*

6. Try tofu ice cream (Tofutti) or low-fat frozen yogurt. These have little fat or cholesterol and contain less sugar than ice cream. Several frozen desserts are sweetened with NutraSweet instead of sugar. The low-fat products may have a higher glycemic index than ice cream.

7. Eat more whole grain breads, cereals, crackers, and pasta.

8. Use the glycemic index only to choose between one carbo and another, not between carbos and fats or proteins. Don't substitute ice cream for potatoes, or sausage for toast.

Moderate Alcohol Use

Alcohol is no longer prohibited for people with diabetes and can be used in moderation, with a few precautions. (Alcohol does not need insulin to be metabolized.)

Alcohol can lower blood sugar. Drinking before dinner may move you into an insulin reaction at the same time that it masks the signs of low blood sugar.

The consequences of intoxication are more significant in diabetics, since getting drunk might lead to skipping a meal or an insulin injection.

On the positive side, in a study of 480 randomly selected Italian and Italian-American adults 73 had overt or borderline diabetes. All 73 were total abstainers or drank wine in small amounts. The remaining 407 drank wine on a regular basis. Other studies have suggested that 1 to 2 ounces of alcohol daily has a protective effect against heart disease. (Abstainers and heavy drinkers had higher incidences of heart disease than moderate drinkers.) Most scientists now agree that this effect is real, although few recommend beginning drinking just to protect your heart. The ADA now approves limited alcohol use with your physician's approval.

Needless to say, the consequences of alcohol abuse are just as serious for the diabetic as for the nondiabetic. Follow these guidelines when you decide to imbibe:

1. Remember to figure the calories of the carbohydrate as well as the alcohol in your drink.

2. Dry wines (most table wines, not dessert wines) have very little carbo in them.

3. Avoid sweet mixers. Use diet soft drinks and diet tonic.

4. You can check the effects of different alcoholic beverages on your metabolism by checking your blood sugar one to two hours after drinking.

Moderate Salt Use

Evidence shows that avoiding salt will lower high blood pressure after it develops. No research has proven that minimizing salt intake will decrease your risk of becoming hypertensive if you do not already have high blood pressure. However, hypertension greatly increases the risk of other complications for a person with diabetes, so prudence argues for restraint with the salt shaker. Less than 2,000 mg a day is low (see Table 3 at end of this chapter for a table listing the salt content of various foods). You can decrease your craving for salt. Begin at home by following these suggestions:

1. Learn to appreciate the flavors of fresh foods without additives.

2. Add only a small amount of salt to the foods you cook.

3. Avoid canned vegetables and other processed and packaged foods, which usually are very high in salt.

4. Use alternative seasonings, such as lemon juice, garlic and onion as well as flavored powders (not salts), other herbs and spices, and wine or flavored vinegars.

5. Limit your use of soy sauce. Even the new low-salt "lite" soy sauce has a lot of salt.

EATING WELL WITH DIABETES

Both of the authors of this book love good food. With creativity and moderation, and using the ideas in this chapter, we have eaten our way healthfully through a variety of restaurants and cuisines. In addition to reading the tips in this chapter, we suggest that you find a nutritionist or dietitian who can tailor some specific diets or menus to your needs and preferences.

Gary's Invisible Diet

My friends are generally not aware that I am thoughtfully monitoring my food and drink intake. For years, I mainly counted only carbohydrates, but more recently I am watching fat more carefully as well. If my schedule of meals will differ from my routine (e.g., Superbowl Sunday, a big dinner dance, a late afternoon movie matinee), I can usually adjust my intake up or down in advance and delay or take extra insulin. A delayed hearty breakfast on Superbowl Sunday will tide me over until the midafternoon party, with its abundant snack foods (eaten mind-fully and in moderation) that become both lunch and supper. The late dinner dance can be taken care of with a later lunch and perhaps some cocktail time appetizers. Popcorn (and maybe chili or a hot dog) in the movie takes care of a potentially very late dinner. Of course, being able to check blood sugars easily helps enormously.

At the end of this chapter, we have listed books and other references we have found helpful, along with some recipes. If you don't have a book that lists food values, we recommend you obtain one; you may be surprised.

Finally, remember that the best way to find out how different foods affect you is to try them and measure their effect on your blood sugar one or two hours after you've eaten. This feedback helps motivate you to change your diet when the tests are high. And it helps you to know the types and amounts of food that are appropriate for you.

Additional Resources: Recipes, Tables, and Books

LOW-FAT, LOW-CHOLESTEROL RECIPES

The following two recipes are from *"Where's the Fat?"* by Martha Wagner: Medical Self Care, Winter, 1984. Note that nonfat and lower fat sour cream are now available in the supermarkets (e.g., Knudsen brand) and nonfat cream cheese is available in selected areas.

ALMOST SOUR CREAM

Yield: 1 cup

Nutrient value per tablespoon: 14 calories, .3 grams fat

1 cup low-fat cottage cheese

2 tablespoons buttermilk or plain, low-fat yogurt

1 tablespoon lemon juice

Combine ingredients in a blender or food processor and blend until smooth.

CREAM CHEESE SUBSTITUTE

Yield: 1 cup

Nutrient value per tablespoon: 24 calories, 1.2 grams fat

1 cup part-skim ricotta cheese

2 tablespoons plain, low-fat yogurt

Combine ingredients in a blender or food processor and puree until smooth. Refrigerate for several hours before serving.

YOLKLESS EGGS

Although these eggs should be made without whole yolks, you can add a small amount of yolk to give the dish a yellow color and improve its texture.

Omelets and fried eggs can be made with yolkless eggs. Whole eggs can also be fried, boiled, or shirred, and the firm yolk removed after cooking. For fried egg whites, separate the whites and fry them as you would a whole egg. For an omelet, separate the whites into a mixing bowl, season with garlic, pepper, and herbs to taste, and mix gently (do not beat them). The pan should be hot enough that a drop of water vaporizes immediately. Use a nonstick pan that is large enough so that the white will cover the bottom and firm up almost immediately throughout. A fat-free nonstick cooking spray can also be used.

For slightly more elaborate (but not necessarily better) scrambled eggs or omelets, you can use the whites and replace each yolk with 1 teaspoon olive or polyunsaturated vegetable oil and 1/2 teaspoon of low-fat dry milk. Yellow food coloring can be added if desired.

Bon appetit!

USEFUL TABLES

Table 1
GLYCEMIC INDEX

Grain Foods		Fruits	
White bread	100	Raisins	93
Whole meal bread	99	Banana	79
Brown rice	90	Orange juice	67
Sweet corn	87	Grapes	62
White rice	83	Apple	53
White spaghetti	66	Pear	47
Whole wheat spaghetti	64	Peach	40
Whole grain rye bread	58	Plum	34
Breakfast cereals		**Sugar**	
Corn Flakes	119	Maltose	152
Weetabix	109	Glucose	138
Shredded Wheat	97	Honey	126
All-Bran	73	Sucrose	86
Root vegetables		Fructose	30
Baked potato (russet)	115	**Dairy products**	
Instant potato	116	Ice cream	52
Boiled potato (new)	81	Yogurt	52
Sweet potato	70	Whole milk	49
		Skim milk	46
Dried peas and beans			
Baked beans (canned)	60		
Dried green peas	56		
Kidney beans	54		
Chick peas	49		
Soy beans (canned)	20		

Note: All foods in this table are standardized against one slice of white bread, assigned a value of 100.

The lower the index, the better: The food is absorbed more slowly.

From Phyllis Crapo, R.D., *Clinical Diabetes*, Jan/Feb 1985, American Diabetes Association.

Table 2
FIBER CONTENT OF SELECTED FOODS

Food	Portion Size	Plant Fiber (grams)
Breads, Cereals, and Starchy Vegetables (cooked/prepared)		
Beans, kidney	½ cup	4.5
Bran (100 percent), cereal	½ cup	10.0
Bread		
Rye	1 slice	2.7
White	1 slice	0.6
Whole grain wheat	1 slice	2.7
Corn, kernels	⅓ cup	2.1
Parsnips	⅔ cup	5.9
Peas	½ cup	5.2
Potatoes, white	1 small	3.8
Rice, brown	½ cup	1.3
Rice, white	½ cup	0.5
Squash, winter	½ cup	3.6
Sweet potatoes	¼ cup	2.9
Fruit (uncooked)		
Apples	1 small	3.9
Banana	½ small	1.3
Blackberries	½ cup	2.6
Grapefruit	½	1.3
Orange	1 small	2.1
Peach	1 medium	1.0
Pineapple	¾ cup	1.3
Strawberries	¼ cup	2.4
Vegetables (cooked unless indicated by plus sign)		
Asparagus	½ cup	1.2
Beans, string	½ cup	1.7
Beets	½ cup	1.5
Broccoli	½ cup	2.6
Carrots	½ cup	2.2
Cauliflower	½ cup	0.9
Cucumbers +	½ cup	0.8
Lettuce +	½ cup	0.5
Squash, summer	½ cup	2.3
Turnips	½ cup	1.3

Note: J. W. Anderson, K. Ward. Long-term effects of high-carbohydrate, high-fiber diets on glucose and lipid metabolism: A preliminary report on patients with diabetes. Diabetes Care 1978, 1:77-82, as adapted for Physician's Guide to Type II Diabetes: Diagnosis and Treatment, American Diabetes Association, 1984.

Table 3
SALT CONTENT OF COMMON FOODS

Fresh/Minimally Processed Foods		Prepared Foods		"Fast Foods"	
1 cup orange juice	2 mg.	1 cup tomato		1 Arby's Turkey	
1 cup apple juice	2 mg.	juice	640 mg.	Sandwich	1,060 mg.
1 cup long-cooking		1 cup Puffed Rice	1 mg.	3 pcs. Arthur	
oatmeal	10 mg.	1 cup Corn		Treacher's Fish	675 mg.
3 ounces ground		Flakes	305 mg.	1 Burger King	
beef	60 mg.	3 ounces corned		Whopper	990 mg.
3 ounces pork	65 mg.	beef	1500 mg.	1 Dairy Queen	
1 cup fresh	5 mg.	1 cup canned		Hot Dog	830 mg.
green bean		green beans	320 mg.	Kentucky Fried	
1 cup frozen		1 cup chicken		Chicken:	
green beans	2 mg.	noodle soup	1050 mg.	3 pieces chicken,	
1 cup whole milk	120 mg.	3 ounces bacon	1400 mg.	mashed potatoes,	
1 large egg	70 mg.	1 dill pickle	1930 mg.	gravy, cole	
1 lemon	1 mg.	1 slice white		slaw	2,285 mg.
1 head Boston		bread	100 mg.	1 McDonald's	
lettuce	15 mg.	cooking oil	0 mg.	Big Mac	1,010 mg.
1 peach	1 mg.	1 cinnamon roll	630 mg.	1 Taco Bell	
8 ounces bluefish	170 mg.	1 tablespoon		Enchirito	1,175 mg.
3 apricots	1 mg.	ketchup	155 mg.		
1 banana	1 mg.	1 cup all-purpose			
1 carrot	35 mg.	flour	2 mg.		
		1 cup self-rising			
		flour	1565 mg.		
		1 beef frank-			
		furter	425 mg.		
		1 tablespoon			
		Italian dressing	250 mg.		
		1 cup instant			
		pudding	335 mg.		
		1 TV chicken			
		dinner	1400 mg.		
		1 olive	165 mg.		
		1 cup baked			
		beans	1000 mg.		

N. Kaplan, M.D., Clinical Diabetes, Mar/Apr, 1984, American Diabetes Association

USEFUL REFERENCES

1. *Health Smart Gourmet Cooking* (A. Hackett, Morningside Publishing Co., One Indian Head Plaza, Suite 600, Nashua, NH, 03060, 1-800-367-2030) has many excellent low-fat recipes and useful preparation and cooking tips, similar to those in his public television cooking series.

2. Any one of Nathan Pritikin's diet books (e.g., *The Pritikin Program for Diet and Exercise*). These books have good recipes for low-fat, low-cholesterol, high-fiber dishes. The full diet is very demanding for some to follow because of the low fat content.

3. The *HCF Guidebook* and *Dr. Anderson's Life-Saving Diet* are two book developed by Dr. James Anderson and colleagues, leading researchers in the effects of such diets. The books are available for purchase from the HCF Diabetes Foundation, P. O. 22124, Lexington, KY 40522, for $8.00 and $7.00 respectively.

4. *Food Values of Portions Commonly Used*, by J. A. T. Pennington and H. N. Church (Harper and Row, 15th edition, 1988) is a handy reference giving grams of fat, carbohydrates, proteins, and other food values.

5. The *New American Diet* (Sonja and William Connor, Simon and Schuster, 1988) and *Eater's Choice: A Food Lovers' Guide to Lower Cholesterol*. (R. and N. Goor, Houghton Mifflin, 1987) are both innovative and useful guides to healthy eating (not specifically for the diabetic).

6. *Fast Foods Facts* (M. J. Franz, 1990) and *Convenience Food Facts* (A. J. Monk and M. J. Franz, 1991) contain useful lists of food values from fast-food chains and name-brand processed foods from 75 companies. Available from CHRONIMED Publishing, P.O. Box 47945, Minneapolis, MN 55391. Ask to be put on the mailing list and request their newsletter, *Living Well With Diabetes*.

7. *Diabetes Forecast*, the monthly magazine of the American Diabetes Association, carries many helpful nutrition articles and recipes. The ADA offers several cookbooks for diabetics. The appendix

at the end of the book gives addresses and telephone numbers for ordering *Forecast* and a catalog of ADA publications.

8. *The Restaurant Companion* (H.S. Warshaw, Surrey Books, Inc., 230 E. Ohio St., Suite 120, Chicago, IL 60611, 1989) provides guidance and tips for restaurant dining in fourteen different cuisines.

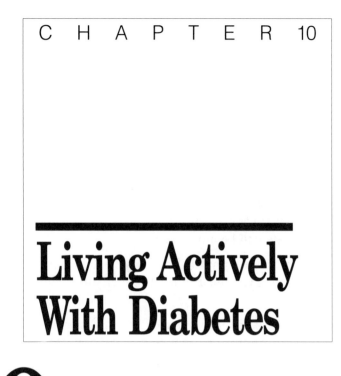

C H A P T E R 10

Living Actively With Diabetes

"O *ne of the good things about diabetes is that it makes a virtue out of enjoying myself physically. The little doctor in the back of my head smiles when I go dancing or swimming, even when I make love. My prescription includes having fun!"*

—Linda

In this chapter, we review the many ways that exercise improves your management of diabetes and reduces the risks of complications. We present an activity questionnaire that helps you assess your present exercise level and plan for improving it. We conclude with guidelines for staying motivated to follow your program.

With so many people jogging and working out, it may seem unnecessary to urge diabetics to exercise. Everybody knows the benefits of staying fit: Exercise decreases your risk of heart disease, lowers high blood pressure, improves general physical fitness, reduces anxiety and depression, and enhances your sense of well-being. As a person with diabetes, however, you enjoy an extra bonus from exercise: It helps you control blood sugar and it lessens the risk of some complications.

215

HOW PHYSICAL ACTIVITY HELPS YOU MANAGE DIABETES

1. Any physical activity lowers your blood sugar by burning it as fuel. You can use exercise to return your levels to normal when tests are high (if BG test is not higher than about 300).

2. Steady exercise for more than twenty minutes enables your muscles to store glucose, further lowering blood sugar after you've stopped exercising. Your body draws on this store when your blood sugar drops too low. When you exercise regularly, your blood sugar levels will be more stable.

3. Consistent physical activity that is moderate or strenuous increases the cell's ability to use insulin. This allows a lower insulin dose.

4. Exercise builds physical fitness, strengthening the heart, circulatory system and lungs, as well as the muscles. This reduces the risk of cardiovascular complications.

5. Exercise is a key to losing or controlling weight and is at least as important as diet.

6. You can neutralize the effects of emotional stress by energetic physical activity.

7. Exercising makes you feel good!

Regular physical activity is a key ingredient of your diabetes control regimen, especially if you want optimal control. Exercise reduces your overall insulin requirement, helps you correct for blood sugar highs, and gives you greater balance in blood sugar levels (once you have adapted to exercising). The cardiovascular gains are especially important to you because, as a diabetic, you have a higher risk of heart and circulatory difficulties. So, in addition to improving your metabolic control, a consistent exercise program makes a heart attack less likely and improves your circulation.

The physical benefits of exercise are echoed at an emotional level. The increased flow of blood and oxygen to the cells and the hormonal shifts that occur when we are physically active lift our spirits. A stressful day at work can be counteracted by a brisk walk or game of tennis. Mild depression may be lightened by an hour of working in the garden or riding a bicycle. When we feel energized, we find it much easier to handle difficult problems and mood swings.

How does all of this magic occur? As soon as we start walking, dancing, swimming, or even swinging our arms, our muscles demand more energy. Blood flow to the muscles increases and soon more oxygen and glucose are moving into the muscle cells. Blood supply to the skin also increases, so the heat generated can be radiated out of the body. As an exercise session progresses, the liver releases additional glucose to fuel the muscles. Fats are also burned to provide further energy.

During physical work or play, insulin and counter-regulatory hormones (adrenalin, growth hormone, glucagon, etc.) interact to ensure an adequate supply of glucose to the cells. Without insulin, the process breaks down in insulin-dependent diabetes. In spite of the activity level, blood sugar will rise steeply and excessive burning of fats will produce ketones if insulin has been omitted. On the other hand, the effectiveness of insulin is increased by exercise. More insulin molecules can connect to the cells and enable glucose to pass through the cell walls.

After you stop exercising, the effects continue to accumulate if you have been playing or working at a moderate to strenuous level. The liver and muscles need to restore their supply of glucose, and they draw it from the bloodstream even when you are resting. This process can go on for several hours following heavy activity. This is why reactions sometimes occur a long time after you've stopped exercising.

Physical activity enables you to lose weight by burning fat and turning glucose into muscle instead of adding more fat. Combining exercise with the proper diet allows a degree of weight control that cannot be obtained by diet alone. In fact, many weight-control programs now recommend at least a week of exercise before you start to diet. The increase in activity level apparently makes appetite control easier.

The power of exercise to relieve stress symptoms is easy to explain: At the most basic level, the stress response is designed to prepare us to act physically. When stressed, we are ready for "fight or flight," so the most natural way to deal with stress is to move vigorously in order to use the hormones and glucose generated by it. This also allows us to release the physical tension that usually accompanies stress, assuming that the exercise includes a relaxed warm-up period.

The short-term effects follow any period of increased physical activity. When you continue the activity long enough to raise your pulse to the target range for your age for fifteen to twenty minutes or more a day, you achieve what is called "the training effect" (discussed later in this chapter). If you do this regularly for a few weeks, you start to enjoy the long-term benefits of exercise. A consistent program of physical training gives you even greater sensitivity to insulin, usually allowing a significant decrease in insulin dosage. Your muscles store more glucose, which is readily available to spontaneously balance low blood sugar. Reactions may become less severe as a result. Your body performs better, your lungs breathe deeper, your heart is stronger, and you feel better. You are living well.

Ernie's Dog Gets Him in Shape

Since completing the first edition of Living Well, I moved back to the city. I now live in a very steep section of the Oakland Hills. Our Siberian Husky needs at least three walks a day, so he's become my aerobic trainer. I've gone from a condition of gasping at the top of our first hill to being able to stride up a whole series of hills and hardly be winded. Last spring I climbed most of the way up the side of Yosemite Valley (on a trail, not the rock wall!) and was still enjoying myself. A age 58 I feel in better shape than I've been since my 30s.

Before we discuss starting or improving your program of physical activity, you may gain some insight into your present activity level by answering the following questions.

MY ACTIVITY PROFILE

1. My typical day includes

   _____ hours of sleep (7-8 hours recommended)

   _____ hours of low activity (riding in or driving a car, reading, watching television, eating, talking while sitting or standing, etc.)

   _____ hours of moderate activity (moderate walking, moderate gardening, mopping, light labor, slow sports like golf or bowling, easy swimming, etc.)

   _____ hours of vigorous activity (rapid walking or running, heavy bicycling, moderate to heavy labor such as digging or carrying heavy objects, climbing stairs, playing tennis or basketball, etc.)

2. At least _____ times a week I increase this to

   _____ hours of moderate activity

   _____ hours of vigorous activity

   _____ This increase of activity happens only on weekends.

   _____ This activity is distributed through the week.

   _____ Although I am usually sedentary, I occasionally have bursts of heavy physical activity.

3. I do some form of stretching or limbering before physical activity.

   _____

   I do stretching as a cool-down after exercise. _____

4. The physical activities I enjoy most are _____

   _____

   Activities I would like to learn are _____

   _____

5. I have the following medical conditions, which need to be considered in designing my activity program:

___Difficulty sensing the signals of an insulin reaction
___Heart disease
___High blood pressure
___Poor circulation
___Retinopahy
___Neuropathy (especially if it involves decreased sensation in the feet)
___I tire quickly
___Back pain (or other muscular or joint discomfort)
___Foot problems
___Other

(If you checked any of the above, you should discuss exercise with your physician. You may need tests to determine the level of activity advisable.)

6. I see the following obstacles to exercising:
___I don't feel I have enough time for it.
___I'm afraid I'll have too many reactions.
___I feel clumsy and uncomfortable with my body.
___I'm bored by physical activities. I prefer using my mind.
___I don't have much energy.
___Other_____

7. I could overcome these obstacles to exercise by_____

_____

8. I would like to increase my level of activity by _____

_____

9. I would like to begin _____

_____

today _____ this week _____this month _____

BEGINNING YOUR ACTIVITY PROGRAM

Without fail, wear a diabetes I.D. bracelet or necklace and inform any gym personnel, coaches, or fellow participants that you have diabetes and may need sugar for an insulin reaction.

We advise you to begin any program of exercise gradually. You need to build strength, endurance, and flexibility so that you will be comfortable exercising. You also have to discover your particular balance between increased activity, insulin, and diet in order to avoid serious reactions. If you have diabetic complications or other physical conditions, you will need to proceed cautiously and with guidance from your doctor. If you are over 35, you should probably have a physical stress test to determine the level of exercise appropriate for you.

Choose activities that you enjoy. You should look forward to your exercise times as positive experiences, not dreaded ordeals. In the following list are several physical activities, ranked according to calories burned. If you have several favorite activities, you will be able to choose among them to deal with changes in weather, mood, and physical state. Although you may prefer to have a partner in exercise, you should also have activities you can do by yourself. If your only physical activity tends to be your work, either on the job or at home, you will gain more benefit from it if you find new ways to enjoy it. Focus on your bodily movements as though they were a dance or a sport. Don't be so fixed on the end product that you ignore your body.

Let Me Count the Ways...

(The category an activity falls into depends on how energetically you do it. An asterisk indicates that activity is good aerobic exercise.)

Light activity (50-200 calories burned per hour)

Stretching	Yoga
Slow t'ai chi chaun	Light housework
Slow walking	Slow social dancing

Moderate Activity (200-400 calories per hour)

Moderate to fast walking*	Bicycling
Gardening	Golf
Mopping	Calisthenics
Tennis (doubles)	Horseback riding
Bowling	Canoeing and rowing
Stationary bicycle*	Trampolining
Swimming*	Square dance or folk dancing*
Ice skating	Fencing
Ping pong and badminton	Aerobic dancing
Making love	Walking up stairs
Slow jogging*	Roller skating
Volleyball	Whirling
Jumping rope*	

Vigorous Activity (400-900 calories per hour)

Digging and shoveling	Bicycle racing
Moderate to rapid jogging*	Football
Hiking*	Racquetball
Chopping wood	Skiing (downhill and cross country)*
Tennis (singles)	Moving furniture
Waterskiing	Ice skating
Running up stairs*	Hill climbing*
Basketball	Squash and handball
	Soccer

You should always warm up before vigorous activity. More importantly, though, you should cool off afterwards. Stretching and limbering muscles for five minutes beforehand and beginning exercise at a moderate pace allows pulse and blood pressure to increase slowly. Cooling down with five or more minutes of slower activity allows your body to return to normal gradually. Neglecting to warm up or cool down can cause risky, abrupt shifts in pulse and blood pressure.

Although any activity helps you become more fit, you will receive the greatest benefit from exercise that requires a fairly steady level of exertion and movement (such as jogging, dancing, or swimming). Stop-and-start activities (such as tennis and volleyball) and static straining (weight lifting) do not build the same level of fitness in your cardiovascular system.

How To Know When You Are Exercising Beyond Your Limit

- If you become faint, dizzy, or nauseated, if you experience severe shortness of breath or tightness or pain in your chest, or if you lose control of your muscles, stop immediately, rest, and discuss these symptoms with your doctor.

- If your pulse or rate of breathing does not return to resting level within three minutes of stopping exercise, you are probably pushing yourself too hard. Take this as a sign to ease up.

- If you are fatigued by moderate activity, and especially if you continue feeling worn out in the hours following, you are doing more than your current condition will support. Cut back in duration or intensity of exercise until you feel stronger. (If this tiredness begins abruptly, it may indicate that you are coming down with a cold or the flu.)

Be sure that you get enough water during exercise. You need regular drinks every fifteen to twenty minutes during strenuous activity.

Exercise and Blood Sugar Levels

Home blood glucose testing and knowledge of your insulin regimen will help you avoid heavy insulin reactions. If you test blood sugar before exercise, ten to fifteen minutes after you stop, and one hour after that, you will see how different types and amounts of activity affect you. (The ten- to fifteen-minute delay after exercising is necessary because sugar from the liver may temporarily raise blood sugar during vigorous activity.) You will have a rough idea of how much exercise it takes to lower a high sugar level and when you need extra food or reduced insulin.

If blood sugar is under 120 before moderate to heavy activity, be sure to eat food that is absorbed quickly (fruit juice, dried fruit, etc.). By trial and error, you will discover how much you need to eat before a given amount of exercise to avoid a reaction or a high blood sugar level. (See Chapter 5, Step 7a for suggestions on changing food and insulin to prepare for extra activity.) Keep in mind when your insulin tends to peak and either eat food if you are exercising at that time or try to match your activity to the times when insulin is not so active. The ideal time for exercise is about one hour after a meal. Blood sugar is at a peak and reactions are less likely to occur then. If you wait two hours or more, you should have a snack before physical activity, unless blood sugar is high.

When you exercise the place where you injected the insulin, the insulin goes to work faster. This can be an advantage if you need to bring down a high blood sugar level, or a disadvantage if you are at a normal level to begin with. If the level is normal, you should avoid your legs as an injection site before a hike, or your racquet arm before a tennis match.

When you exercise fairly heavily or over a long period (over an hour), your blood sugar will continue to decrease after you stop. The muscles and liver are replenishing their stores. You may need a larger meal or extra snacks to avoid reactions in the hours following a time of high or extended exertion.

Keep in mind the overall interaction between insulin, diet, and activity. You can vary any one or a combination of these factors to compensate for high blood sugar levels or changes in routine. This allows you a high degree of flexibility while maintaining good metabolic control.

If blood sugar is high (around 250-300 mg/dl), exercise is not an effective way to lower it. Vigorous activity may even cause blood sugar to rise because not enough insulin is on board to utilize the blood sugar, and the exercise is releasing adrenalin, which also raises the blood sugar. If ketones are present, they will also increase. Extra insulin or less food are the best ways to reduce very high blood sugar levels.

Similarly, if you are ill, you should avoid all but the mildest activities. Your body needs energy to deal with the stress of the illness. Exercise only adds to this physical stress and may even worsen the condition.

The Training Effect

The greatest benefits of exercise occur when you regularly reach the training effect. This is achieved through sustained activity that raises your pulse to your target level for at least twenty minutes. If you do this at least three times a week (every other day), both your heart and your metabolic system will function better, assuming you have no major diabetic complications.

You have a built-in meter right at your fingertips for measuring the effectiveness and the safety of any type of physical activity. Count the number of heartbeats you can feel at your wrist or throat (just above the collarbone toward the center of your throat) for fifteen seconds, multiply by 4, and you have your pulse rate. Do this when resting and then during and immediately following exercise. The following table gives the meaning of different pulse rates, in terms of exercise intensity.

Listen To Your Heart

Pulse Rate (beats per minute)	Degree of Exertion You Feel	Comments
60-80	Very, very light	Of little value as exercise
80-100	Very light	Useful if condition is very poor
100-120	Moderate	Intensity just right
120-140	Somewhat hard	
140-160	Very hard	Stop! unless you are an athlete in top condition

Those of you reluctant to stop and measure your pulse can simply use the degree of exertion that feels right to you as your guide. If you are unable to talk to a fellow exerciser, you are probably overdoing it. If you work in the moderate to somewhat hard range, you will probably be at the level you need.

Another indication of your ability to handle exercise is the time it takes for your pulse to return to your resting rate after exertion. Measure it after you have been sitting quietly for fifteen minutes, move vigorously for as long as it takes to get your pulse over 120, then rest and measure your pulse again at one-minute intervals. If it takes more than three minutes to return to your resting rate, you are in poor shape and need to proceed cautiously with your exercise program. A more precise way of assessing your condition is to undergo an endurance or stress test at your doctor's office or at the local YMCA or YWCA.

If you have been fairly sedentary, you may find that even relatively mild activity will bring your pulse up to a high level quickly. Your body is out of condition, and your heart has to work hard to handle any increased exercise. Recognize that your limits will gradually expand, and don't push yourself too hard. Twelve to twenty minutes a day at a pulse rate of 100 to 120 is a good beginning. (If you are over 60 and have not been very active, start with five minutes a day.) Stay at this level for a couple of weeks, and increase the duration and intensity of activity only when you feel your endurance growing.

As you get in better condition, you will find that you are exerting yourself harder before you reach the same pulse rate. The flight of stairs that left you breathless and your heart pounding a few weeks ago will be handled with ease. *If you don't experience improved endurance, be sure to discuss this with your physician.*

As you experience progress in endurance and performance, you will be able to gradually raise your sights. If your doctor approves, you can increase the duration and intensity of exercise every two or three weeks until you are at your peak. For a younger person without complications, peak performance would allow a pulse rate of 140 to 160 beats per minute for sessions of thirty to sixty minutes. It can take up to six months to reach this level of conditioning, depending on where you start. If you are older, a lower pulse rate goal should be set, depending on age.

Pulse Rate by Age		
Age	Recommended pulse	Pulse rate if you have history of heart disease, not to exceed:
20	130-170	150
30	124-162	143
40	117-153	137
45	114-149	134
50	111-145	131
55	107-140	128
60	104-136	120
65	101-132	113

How Often Do You Need to Exercise?

Three workout sessions a week can be enough to build conditioning. However, if you have diabetes, you benefit from the blood sugar lowering effects as well. Ideally, you should include some physical activity in your schedule every day. This regularity helps you maintain good blood sugar levels consistently. You can't always meet this ideal, but fortunately you can use your skill at varying the ingredients of your regimen to deal with varying levels of activity. Diet or insulin dosage can be tailored to the kind of day you plan. A few more units of insulin or smaller meals will help maintain balance on the sitting-around-and-reading-or-watching-television kinds of days.

What If You Have an Active Job?

Your work may be vigorous enough to keep you physically fit without further exercise. It depends upon the degree of exertion and the variety of movements you use. If your pulse stays in the range of 100 to 140 for extended periods during the day, you are working at a level that satisfies conditioning requirements. However, if your pulse is usually below 100 even when active on the job, you may need to add more active movement. If your job keeps you moving in the same repetitive patterns, you may need limbering and loosening exercises to avoid sore muscles and maintain full flexibility.

GUIDELINES FOR DEVELOPING AN ACTIVITY PROGRAM YOU WILL FOLLOW

1. Build on the physical activities you already enjoy doing. Your exercise program may take several hours a week for the rest of your life. Start with the activities that give you real pleasure, and then learn some of the ones you've always wished you could do. Avoid boredom by using several different forms of active exercise.

2. If you feel short of time, do things simultaneously: socialize and exercise at the same time (friends don't always have to sit down!); ride the exercise bicycle while watching television or listening to music; hold business discussions as you walk.

3. Keep a balance between developing more endurance and staying comfortable. You need time to strengthen your heart and muscles and to learn how to adjust diet and insulin to your new level of exercise. If you go too fast, pain and insulin reactions may discourage you from continuing. This is especially important if you are over 35, if you have any signs of heart trouble, or if other complications have started to develop.

4. Use your knowledge of changing diet and insulin dosage to prepare for increased physical activity. You are probably better off having a few high blood sugar tests from eating a little more than you need than risking serious reactions. Feedback from your tests will soon tell you how much is enough. Exercise beginning thirty to sixty minutes after a meal is least likely to cause reactions. If activity comes two or more hours after eating, you should have a snack unless blood sugar is over 150 mg/dl.

5. If you have a distaste for exercise because you are a "mental" type, use the "inner-sports" approach. Techniques such a visualization, affirmation and meditation help many people understand the strong relationship between mind and body and reinforce motivation to exercise. Another possibility is to keep an exercise log and calculate your progress.

6. If you are anxious about exercise because of limiting physical conditions, ask your doctor for guidelines to ensure safety. You might consider joining a class specifically designed for people with physical limitations. Your YMCA, March of Dimes, ADA chapter, or adult-education school may have a program taught by someone trained to help you exercise safely and monitor your special condition. Organizations for the visually handicapped may also be of help.

7. If you are reluctant to move because everyone will see how clumsy and awkward you are, try starting with walking. It's hard to look so clumsy while walking that anyone notices, and you can use walking exercise to develop your sense of grace. The trick is to pay attention to your body as you walk. Keep your attention turned to the sensations in your feet, legs, hips, arms, back, and shoulders. Let go of any tightness you notice. Then apply this same awareness to any form of motion. You are likely to find any awkwardness decreasing as you learn to be conscious of your body and release its tensions.

8. If competitive activities make you anxious, avoid them. The stress they create for you will tend to offset the benefits of the exercise. (Others may find the spirit of competition necessary to maintain motivation and avoid boredom.)

9. If you exercise outside, do it away from busy streets. Deeper breathing isn't so healthful when the air you breathe is full of carbon monoxide.

10. A great workbook may help you get motivated to develop an easy and specific plan for a walking program. It's oriented toward weight loss but is useful for anyone. It's the *Walking Off Weight Workbook* by Robert J. Sweetgall (Creative Walking, Inc., P.O. Box 50296, Clayton, MO 63105, 1-800-762-9255).

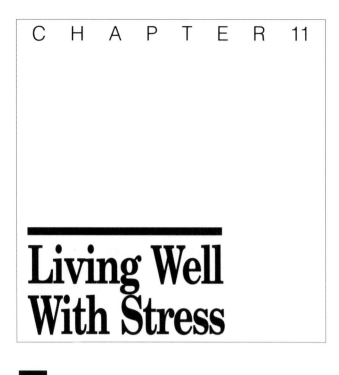

C H A P T E R 11

Living Well
With Stress

In recent years, a distressing amount of information has been spread about the effects of stress on health. As people with diabetes, we have reasons to take special interest in the subject of stress:

• Simply having diabetes generates stress-inducing events.

• Either physical or emotional stress can play havoc with our blood sugar levels.

• Chronic stress can contribute to the development of diabetic complications.

These three facts alone make an effective stress-management program a high priority for anyone with diabetes. If you follow such a program, you will be stabilizing your blood sugar levels by reducing the effect of stress on your metabolism. You will be lowering the risk of developing complications, and you will find it easier to live well with diabetes as you neutralize the distress of having it.

Let's examine the three ways that stress affects diabetes.

Simply having diabetes generates stressful events.

How many simple events become stressful for us because we have diabetes? "Sorry, dinner's going to be a bit late." "I'm afraid your bag got put on another plane." "Looks like that blister on your foot has gotten a little infected." "No, there's no drugstore open on Sunday here." Our sense of security depends upon an amazing number of routines functioning smoothly. We are vulnerable to happenings that to others may be trivial.

In almost every hour of the waking day, we must consider some aspect of our self-care and we may be confronted with a significant diabetes problem to solve. Even our sleeping hours may be shattered by the shaking cold sweat of an insulin reaction (itself an event of powerful physical stress).

These day-to-day stresses of diabetes can build strong feelings of guilt and anxiety because they remind us of a deeper fear: the fear of diabetic complications. No matter how much we may try to forget the possibility of blindness, kidney failure, or heart disease, our mind remembers at some level that we are at risk. Anything that suggests this risk becomes a source of further stress.

Now is probably an excellent time to practice some stress management. Check yourself to see how you responded to the statements you just read. What changes can you detect in your body? Do you feel edgy, tense, nervous, suddenly tired? How did your mind respond? Did you want to stop reading, to deny that you are at risk?

Close your eyes and say to yourself slowly, "I am learning to take better care of myself. I am reducing the risks." Let the words relax you as you repeat them several times. If any other words try to deny what you are affirming, just hear them as static.

This illustrates one way of reducing stress: working to replace the thoughts that trigger it with more reassuring thoughts.

Either physical or emotional stress can play havoc with our blood sugar levels.

Diabetes gives us added sources of stress. And, adding insult to injury, diabetics are more vulnerable to its effects. Physiologically, the stress response is a powerful shift in hormone levels. It can raise, and sometimes lower, blood sugar levels to two or three times the normal level. Ironically, a botched and painful drawing of blood by an incompetent lab technician can result in an artificially high test result because of the emotional stress. Similarly, a bad scare while driving or a frustrating put-down by the boss can send blood sugar soaring. Many so-called brittle diabetics are probably simply people who don't know how to manage the stress in their lives.

Similarly, physical stresses such as infections, wounds or burns are likely to have a powerful effect on metabolism, raising both blood sugar and ketone levels. These high levels, if uncontrolled, slow down healing and can result in medical emergencies and hospitalization. The skills of blood glucose testing and adjusting insulin dosage can be lifesavers when we suffer severe physical stress.

Chronic stress can contribute to the development of diabetic complications.

High blood sugar levels are usually thought to be the primary cause of complications, but there is growing evidence that stress also plays a role here. Heart disease, for instance, is strongly associated with poorly managed stress in the general population. With diabetes, high levels of stress hormones may contribute to such conditions as retinopathy. Stress definitely is a factor in hypertension (high blood pressure), which in turn contributes to the development of a number of complications. Clearly, effective management of stress is an important component in any program to reduce the risk of complications.

Poorly managed stress has a major impact on the health of everyone— not just the health of diabetics. Many books, magazines, television shows, and classes have been detailing this impact and offering suggestions for handling stress. Stress is believed to contribute to heart disease, hypertension, and cancer. Although other factors also play a role in any of these conditions, reducing your stress level is likely to increase your chances of living well.

UNDERSTANDING THE STRESS RESPONSE

Stress is an inherent part of living. When a change in our environment demands something of us, our bodies react, preparing to meet the demand. There are similarities in this reaction no matter what the external stimulus (called the stressor): a threat of physical attack, an emotional blow, a joyous event, a burst of energetic activity, or an actual injury or illness. The stress response is our body's attempt to maintain or restore healthful conditions in all our physical systems.

You can appreciate the great value of the stress response simply by remembering the last time you had a strong insulin reaction. You probably felt shaky and nervous, your pulse speeded up, your blood pressure increased, and you may have become sweaty and emotional. These outward cues were responses to the physical emergency of low blood sugar. The adrenal hormones released as the result of this physical stress caused the symptoms you experienced. (They also signaled the liver to release glucose and glucagon into your blood stream in an attempt to correct the low blood sugar.) The same hormones also tend to neutralize the effectiveness of insulin so it will not lower blood sugar any further.

If you had become unconscious, this automatic system might have been enough to bring you around, if you were lucky. The body treats this situation as an emergency because the brain needs a certain level of glucose to function effectively and may be damaged if blood sugar falls to very low levels.

Now, if the stressor was the threat of a mugging or negative criticism from a fellow worker or a bad fall, you would probably experience the same stress response. The hormones flow, blood sugar goes up, insulin becomes less effective, and you are ready for "fight or flight." Your energy is mobilized for an all-out effort.

You can see what a negative effect this mobilization has on metabolic control, unless the appropriate response to the situation is a major physical event. Your pancreas is unable to contribute enough additional insulin to burn all that extra blood sugar stimulated by the stress. Your next test would be high, and if you didn't know about the effects of stress, you might be shaking your head in puzzlement, saying, "But I didn't eat any more than usual!" You might not even be conscious of the source of distress, and the symptoms of the stress response may sometimes be subtle enough to escape notice, though blood sugar still rises.

Ernest's Traffic with Stress

I'm generally very polite and restrained, earnest even, but in traffic I used to express myself rather emphatically when other drivers treated me unkindly...until the last and absolutely final time I ever made an obscene gesture on the freeway. I was chased down Interstate 5 through Seattle, onto city streets, and back to the freeway for seven miles before I finally ditched my offended pursuer. I did my best to meditate while weaving in and out of traffic, but I still ended up with blood sugar at 500 mg/dl by the time I got home.

The threat doesn't have to be so real, though, to raise my blood sugar. A number of times I have found that my emotional participation in a movie I'm watching has been enough to produce similar increases.

On the other hand, there have been times when blood sugar has gone down to a reaction level after I got angry and expressed it strongly.

One other aspect of the stress response has a special importance for people with diabetes. Both physical and emotional stress can have a powerful effect on blood ketone levels. In some adolescents, ketones have increased tenfold during family arguments.

Stress does not stop with these effects that relate directly to diabetes. Your muscles tense, preparing for action and expression. When you are unable to release this tension, headaches, back pain, and other muscular disorders may occur. Your digestive system becomes involved, with changes in secretion of stomach acids, digestive hormones, and the muscle tone of the alimentary canal. Blood fat and cholesterol levels increase to provide additional energy for action. Pulse and blood pressure increase. The whole body participates in the stress response. If the cycle is not completed by action, the tension, hormones, glucose, fats, and other stress products stay at unnaturally high levels. If the stress is chronic and poorly managed, your health suffers.

From the point of view of its stress-producing activity, it is immaterial whether the agent or situation we face is pleasant or unpleasant; all that counts is the intensity of the demand for readjustment or adaptation...[We need] to distinguish between distress, which is always unpleasant, and the general concept of stress, which...also includes the pleasant experiences of joy, fulfillment, and self-expression.

—Hans Selye in *Stress Without Distress*

Although stress has powerful effects on diabetes control, it still is not a major subject of research. On the basis of existing studies, it is not easy to predict whether stress is more likely to raise or lower blood sugar in any given person with diabetes.

This gap in scientific knowledge is based, in part, on the difficulty of doing reliable stress research. (One study in the late 1940s would probably be rejected today by research review committees on the grounds of cruelty. In it, the doctor tested his subjects' blood sugar level and then berated them for being weak and spineless for controlling their diabetes so poorly. Then he tested again and found higher blood sugar. He apologized.)

Although scientists are not totally certain about anything concerning stress and diabetes, you do not have to wait for their conclusions on the subject. Armed with your blood glucose test kit, your urine ketone test strips, and your logs, you can do the research that is most important to you: Determine how stress affects you as an individual. (Apparently the impact of stress is highly individual.)

Note distressing or exciting events and periods; study your test results in terms of these events. See if there is a difference in blood sugar level during a week when you are depressed and during a week when you are happier than usual. What happens after a quarrel or a frightening episode? The following list of questions can help you discover how stress affects your diabetes.

Some Questions to Guide Your Personal Research on Stress

1. Does stress seem to have much effect on your blood sugar level? If so, is your blood sugar level increased or decreased?

2. Does the type of emotion aroused influence the direction or amount of change in blood sugar?

3. What difference do you see between short, intense moments of distress and long drawn-out episodes? What impact do you find from stress that extends for days or weeks at a time?

4. Is the effect on blood sugar level different when you express feelings fully rather than holding them in? (One classic study found blood sugar in one woman unaffected after she became angry and hit her mother-in-law over the head. We hope that more modest forms of expression prove adequate!)

5. Do you have positive tests for ketones in your urine after stressful incidents? If so, when?

6. How do any attempts to cope with stress through self-gratification (such as overeating, drinking, and not exercising) disrupt control?

7. What overall pattern do you see in the ways you respond to stress?

As you understand more about how stress affects your control of diabetes, you will be better equipped to handle it. You will know that you need to check your blood sugar level after certain kinds of experiences to see whether you need extra insulin. You will know whether you need to modify your insulin dose during times of increased (or decreased) stress. And you will have evidence of the kinds of stressful experiences you need to learn to manage more effectively.

Recognizing the Symptoms of Stress

Acute symptoms	Chronic symptoms
Pounding heart, rapid pulse	General irritability
Trembling, shaky	Depression
Dry throat and mouth	Easily fatigued
Hard to concentrate	Loss of appetite
Change in blood sugar level	Anxiety
Emotional and physical tension	Insomnia
Sweating	Missed menstrual periods
Easily startled	Nervous tics
Diarrhea or frequent urination	Stuttering
Indigestion	Migraines
Tension headaches	Chronic muscular pains
Compulsive eating	Nightmares
	More accidents and mistakes than usual

—adapted from *The Stress of Life* by Hans Selye (McGraw-Hill, 1976)

Some of us are more aware of feelings and physical sensations and have no difficulty spotting the signs of stress. If this is not true for you, you may need to spend time developing more awareness of this side of your life. Ignoring the effects of stress does not decrease the impact of stress. If you know when stress is building, you are better able to do something about it. With more awareness of your body, you are also able to detect the onset of an insulin reaction sooner.

At times, you may mistake an insulin reaction for a general stress response, or vice versa, because the symptoms overlap. You may have some clear signs of low blood sugar: blurred or double vision, tingling, or metallic taste on the tongue. If in doubt (and if you cannot test your blood at the time), eat a moderate amount of something sweet and see if the symptoms decrease at all.

DOING SOMETHING ABOUT STRESS

There are four main styles of managing stress:

1. Reduce the frequency of stressful incidents by

    a. Making changes in your family, social, or work situation.

    b. Changing beliefs and emotional patterns that trigger stress for you.

    c. Gaining skills that allow you to function more effectively.

    d. Preparing for events likely to be distressing.

2. Reduce the intensity of your stress response by

    a. Learning to relax

    b. Meditating

    c. Praying

    d. Using biofeedback

3. Put the stress response to work by becoming more active physically.

4. Decrease your consumption of stimulants.

As with other aspects of diabetes regimens, coping with stress is a highly individual matter. Vulnerability to stress, the level of arousal, the effectiveness of any particular coping technique all vary from person to person. Fortunately, there are many different approaches to stress management, so you can find at least one that works for you.

The only formula is this: Whatever you do should not increase your stress level. Find an approach that suits you.

1. **Reduce the frequency of stressful incidents**
   a. Make changes in your family, social, or work situation.

You may find it easiest to act on your environment, demanding or requesting changes in the people and conditions that produce stress for you. Or, for the less assertive, you may be able to withdraw from whatever is distressing to you. For instance, you might have a doctor who doesn't listen to you or who tries to motivate you with fear. You could say how that approach affects you and ask for changes. If your physician doesn't respond, or if you choose to avoid a direct interaction, you could change doctors.

   b. Change beliefs and emotional patterns that trigger stress for you.

You may prefer to work on yourself, using the source of stress to show you the areas of your personality that need change. With the same insensitive doctor, you might discover that the root of your stress is a belief such as "No one thinks anything I say is important." By neutralizing this belief, you would reduce your stress and probably find it easier to speak with more strength.

Similarly, you could work with the feeling of stifled anger triggered when an authority figure ignores you. By learning to express or become detached from such responses, you gain power to use the energy they release. (See Chapter 14 for more on working with beliefs and feelings.)

   c. Gain skills that allow you to function more effectively.

Often the source of distress is a sense of inadequacy that can be corrected by learning to perform tasks that are important to us. This might involve skills of learning, working, relating or even of simply enjoying life. You might overcome your physician's resistance to listening by taking a workshop in assertiveness training or communication skills (assuming this was not the only relationship in which you had difficulty getting your point across).

d. Prepare for events likely to be distressing.

We often do this negatively, imagining everything that can possibly go wrong, sometimes in great detail. This skill of visualization can be turned into a positive resource in the following way: Relax deeply and then imagine living through the event. Imagine yourself performing with calm, strength, and clarity, no matter what others do. Go through the experience in detail several times if you see yourself faltering. Then forget about it so you won't try to use the visualization as a map when you get to the actual event. Real life calls for spontaneous, not rehearsed, action.

2. **Reduce the intensity of your stress response by learning to relax**

Your body knows how to relax, but sometimes your mind forgets to use this essential skill. When you practice it in the midst of a distressing incident, you can lessen the physical impact of the event. When you forget to relax until afterward, you still benefit from releasing the tensions that developed under stress. A relaxed body deals with stress more effectively and also provides the best conditions for creative problem solving. Some studies have also indicated that people with diabetes who regularly practice relaxation improve their metabolic control. It also just feels better to be relaxed!

There is a wonderful variety of relaxation techniques: visualization, massage, music, autogenics, meditation, prayer, and biofeedback. If you learn several ways of relaxing, you will have one to use no matter what external situation you have to face. (This chapter contains several examples of relaxation techniques.)

One tip: Whatever relaxation techniques you choose, practice them while sitting, standing, or moving, as well as while lying down. It is important to learn that you can lose tension in any position, especially since it is more likely to strike when you're up and about.

Visualization involves using mental imagery in any sense mode (not just visual) to produce relaxation. Examples are imagining warm water flowing gently across tense muscles; imagining each breath carrying tension out of your body; or imagining warm light moving through your body. Your body releases tension in response to this visualization process.

Autogenics, on the other hand, uses words to instruct the body to relax. By telling yourself that your arms and legs are becoming heavier, and then warmer, you are suggesting that the results of relaxation are beginning to take effect. As you repeat the phrases, your body responds by relaxing deeply. Physicians in Europe have reported decreased insulin requirements in diabetics who regularly practice autogenics.

Massage can relax tense muscles, as well as lead to a sense of well-being. Self-massage of temples, neck, shoulders, feet, and calves can relieve tightness, stiffness, or even pain. Learning specific acupressure points for massage is another way to help relax.

Quiet and peaceful music can be used to shape special periods of relaxation and is also effective as background sound. (In fact, relaxing music might help you as you work with this book.) Our bodies respond to excess noise with tension, but they tend to relax when the sounds around us are tranquil. (The resource list at the end of the chapter lists records and tapes that can be used.)

Meditation is a centuries-old means of contacting inner sources of strength and calmness. The physical effects of meditation have been shown to quiet the ravages of stress in our bodies.

Prayer may be seen as a meditation of words directing awareness to a sense of unity and connectedness. Some envision their words being received by a deity; others imagine them simply joining the wholeness of the universe.

3. Put the stress response to work by becoming more active physically

Since the stress response is designed to prepare us for maximum physical activity, exercise is ideally suited to using the physical changes produced by stress in a positive way. Try running up and down stairs after you learn you will not get that hoped-for-promotion. Jog or dance after a quarrel with your lover. Thirty to sixty minutes of exercise at a moderate to brisk level will use the adrenalin and start to bring down the blood sugar. (If you have very high blood sugar because of stress, you may need extra insulin.)

4. Decrease your consumption of stimulants

Caffeine in coffee and tea and nicotine in cigarettes, along with their other negative effects, can add to stress. Although they are advertised as calming, their actual effect may be just the opposite.

Any one of these techniques for managing stress will benefit your health. If you have a fairly stressful life, you may need to combine several of them to cope with the demands on you. Find the right combination for you, and be gentle in its application. Don't make stress management one more source of stress in your life.

RELAXATION EXERCISES

First, remember to practice relaxation in a variety of situations— while sitting, standing, and moving as well as lying down. You can relax anywhere, not just when you're flat on your back. (If you are usually tense, though, you may want to start learning to relax when lying down, with your eyes closed.)

Give up the waste of time calling *waiting*. No matter where you are, you can use those in-between times to let go of tensions and notice what's happening with your body. As long as you don't start snoring, no one will notice or care what you are doing.

Breathe Away Tensions

Begin by just noticing how you are breathing. What part of your torso are you using? How deep or shallow is your breathing? How fast?

Then, focus on the feeling of air moving in and out of your nostrils for a minute. Follow the air down into your lungs and feel your chest and stomach expand and contract with each breath.

Focus now on each exhalation, imagining that the air is carrying tension out of your body. If you are alone, sigh or hum gently with each breath.

242

Finally, focus on each inhalation, imagining new energy coming into your body with the air.

Visualize With Any or All of the Senses

A simple visualization to use for relaxation is to imagine yourself immersed in a sensory bath—fragrant, warm breezes; tropical showers; glowing light; gentle, natural sounds . . . . Sense warm water and breezes flowing over each muscle of your body, even through the muscles, opening and relaxing them.

An alternative visualization: Let your mind return you to a specific time when you felt happy and deeply relaxed. Relive the event in as much detail as you can recall.

Talk Your Body Into Relaxing

When our minds talk, our bodies listen. European doctors have created a whole discipline of relaxation on the basis of this simple truth. Called autogenic training, this approach uses repeated phrases to suggest to the body that it is experiencing relaxation...and it does.

Repeat each phrase slowly (and silently) five or six times:

> "My right arm is growing heavier."
> "My left arm is growing heavier."
> "My right leg is growing heavier."
> "My left leg is growing heavier."
> "My right arm is growing warmer."
> (and so on through the other limbs).

Meditate

Among the numerous approaches to meditation, one of the easiest to learn is called mindfulness. With this, you step back from the constant flow of thoughts and sensations and simply watch the parade.

Find a posture you can maintain comfortably without moving for ten to twenty minutes. Balance your body so you are not leaning forward or backward or to the side. (Or lie down if you can stay awake.)

Begin with awareness of the breath passing through your nostrils, and use this sensation as an anchor. Each breath can be a reminder that all you have to do is watch the flow of thoughts, feelings, perceptions, and body sensations. Just watch, without commenting on or judging what you see.

Naturally you forget to "just watch" and you become immersed time and again in the process of thinking, feeling, and so on. You forget even the simple task of sensing each breath. But soon your breath itself reminds you that you can detach and step back again.

You move back and forth between just watching and marching along in the parade of your mind. Then gradually the periods of watching grow longer and the mind grows quieter.

RESOURCES FOR STRESS MANAGEMENT

Books on Relaxation

Herbert Benson, *The Relaxation Response*, Avon, 1975

Patricia Carrington, *Freedom in Meditation*, Anchor Books, 1978

Daniel Girdano and George Everly, *Controlling Stress and Tension*, Prentice-Hall, 1979

Joseph Levine, *A Gradual Awakening*, Doubleday, 1984

Hans Selye, *Stress Without Distress*, Signet, 1975

Norman Shealy, *90 Days to Self-Health*, Dial, 1978

Music to Help You Relax

Gregorian Chant and other early church music (before Baroque)

William Ackerman, *Passages*, Windham Hill Records

Brian Eno, *Music for Airports* or *Plateaux of Mirrors*, ECM

Steve Halprin, *Spectrum Suite*, SRI Records

Georgia Kelly, *Seapeace*, Global Pacific

Environments (natural sounding records—waves, bird song, country streams, and the like) Cyntonic Research, 175 5th Ave., New York, NY

Guided-Relaxation Tapes

Emmett Miller, *Letting Go of Stress* and *Health and Wellness*

Classes on Stress Management

Your local chapter of the American Diabetes Association may offer or know of a stress-management class especially designed for people with diabetes.

YMCA and high school or college adult-education programs usually have general stress-management classes.

Section IV
SUPPORT FOR LIVING WELL

Living Well With Your Medical Team

Of all the chronic medical conditions, diabetes probably has the most sophisticated, well-developed team of health professionals dedicated to helping you learn about and manage the disease. There is even an American Association of Diabetes Educators (AADE) with several thousand members. Membership includes a wide variety of professionals all interested and involved in working with diabetes. Who are they?

DIABETES HEALTH PROFESSIONALS

Physicians

Most likely, your primary physician is either a family physician or an internist. The physician may or may not have special interest or expertise in diabetes. There are also subspecialists—endocrinologists and diabetologists—who have special training in diabetes. Any of these physicians can help you live well with your diabetes. You may find one who is more responsive to your individual needs, more knowledgeable about the options available, more willing to work with you, than another. These qualities may well be more related to the physician's personal characteristics than to training. You have the right to choose a physician with whom you have a mutually rewarding relationship. You need not feel guilty if you decide to change doctors because you want a better relationship.

If complications develop, your physician may refer you (or you may ask for a recommendation) to a specialist or subspecialist in the area of your complication: for skin problems, a dermatologist; for nerve problems, a neurologist; for kidney problems, a nephrologist; for problems with digestion or bowels, a gastroenterologist or neurologist (since these problems in a diabetic are usually due to neuropathy); and for eye problems, an ophthalmologist. We recommend that you see an ophthalmologist at least once a year on a preventive basis.

Podiatrists and Dentists

Diabetes can affect you from head to toe. It is wise to have regular (yearly, and more often, if recommended) preventive maintenance on your teeth and gums and your feet. You should be sure that your dentist and podiatrist are aware that you have diabetes. It will affect the signs and symptoms they look for and the kind of treatment they may give you.

Diabetes Educators

In this category, we include nurses, nurse educators, nurse practitioners, dietitians, nutritionists, patient educators, and exercise specialists. Diabetes educators know that the knowledge, skills and attitudes involved in living well with diabetes require someone who is well trained to help the patient learn them. The nurse or patient educator may teach most areas and may refer you to a dietitian if you need detailed information in the areas of food, nutrition and weight. An exercise specialist can help you design a program of sports or exercises suited to your level of fitness.

The AADE has recently instituted a program of certification for diabetes educators. Educators who pass a comprehensive exam become Certified Diabetes Educators and are entitled to put the initials "CDE" after their names. A CDE is likely to be well informed about the latest and best methods of diabetes management, although many excellent diabetes educators are not certified.

Psychologists, Psychiatrists, Counselors and Other Psychotherapists

These professionals are available to help you with crises or difficult changes that you wish to make in your life. They can help you overcome resistance to following the diabetes regimen you choose, if you need more than the techniques presented in this book. They are also very useful in helping you deal with the emotional and the problem-solving aspects of crises like the onset of complications. You may be able to find someone who specializes in diabetes or other chronic illnesses through your local chapter of American Diabetes Association. (See Chapter 13 for more on the times when professional psychological support may be needed, as well as some powerful sources of lay support.)

Pharmacists

Pharmacists an be extremely helpful in providing information on insulin, other medications and their effect on your diabetes, and the selection and use of a wide variety of diabetes products.

WORKING WITH THE TEAM

The idea of a team implies coordination of rules and responsibilities to accomplish a mutually shared goal. You are the focus, and the team's general goal is helping you to live well with diabetes.

It is your responsibility to convey to individuals on the team your needs, concerns, questions and problems. As health professionals ourselves, we urge you to speak up

• when you do not understand something you are told.

• when too much is being told you at once.

• when you think you will have difficulty carrying out a recommendation.

- when you may not agree with something you are told to do.

- when you want to know if there are alternatives to the plan recommended.

Most health professionals prefer that you voice lack of understanding or disagreement from the start rather than not say anything because you may feel awkward or embarrassed. Otherwise, you're both wasting time. Health professionals realize that *you* make the ultimate decisions about your care, and they want you to understand their recommendations fully and be willing to follow them.

It is the health professional's responsibility to communicate clearly to you about your care and the options available to you. They should use words you understand, speak slowly enough for you to follow, and write down or provide printed information about their recommendations. They should outline the risks and benefits of alternative courses of action and explain any side effects of recommended tests, medications, procedures, or treatments.

As you read this book and work with members of the diabetes team, you may wish to bring this book with you. With the health professional, go over parts of the book that are particularly relevant to you at the time, ask questions about what might not be clear to you, and show them this chapter, if desired. In particular, you may wish to show them the special note in the Preface.

The basic tool of your diabetes care team is communication. We hope that this book will help support the communication between you and the members of your team.

Living Well With Other Diabetics

"I *always felt lonely and a little weird, like I was the only diabetic in the world who lied to her doctor or ate lemon meringue pie. The only thing worse than my guilt was my depression over feeling so out of control. I didn't think anyone could understand what I was up against, until I went—not very willingly—to a diabetes support group. For the first time, I got to talk to people who were struggling with the same issues that had me down. They taught me I could do something to get myself under control."*

—Jean

CREATING A DIABETES SUPPORT NETWORK

Diabetes is a demanding companion that tends to isolate us from others. Our friends and relations may have little understanding of the frustrations and challenges we face. We may believe we would only bore them with the countless details of regimen we stay aware of every day. We need a special quality of support that depends upon living knowledge of diabetes: support for coping with our feelings, support for solving the many practical questions we need answered, support for improving our ability to follow our complex regimen.

Contact with others who are attempting to live well with diabetes is a vital ingredient in our program of self-care.

Support from other people with diabetes is especially important when you decide to improve your level of management. The experiences, practical knowledge, and understanding of someone else who has gone through this process make the path much easier. Others can help you see when you are trying to move too fast or when you are forgetting important aspects of regimen. They can offer encouragement and practical tips. This level of support is a beautiful complement to the direction you obtain from your medical team.

Support is especially important when diabetes is first diagnosed or when complications first appear. These are times of crisis when we may be filled with strong feelings and countless questions. Others with diabetes can help us deal with these challenges and learn the lessons of living well.

Those who are close to us need support as well. Being the mate or parent of someone with diabetes has its own unique demands. Just ask a person who has found a loved one unconscious or who watches one of us consistently overeating. Our close friends can learn from and be encouraged by others with diabetes and their families.

Anyone with diabetes may encounter problems that require professional mental health assistance. Our support system may be weak, or the particular challenges we meet may require the aid of someone with professional training. Some of the signs of needing to see a psychotherapist, counselor, or social worker include

1. Chronic depression.

2. Repeated self-destructive behavior such as "forgetting" insulin, going on frequent eating binges, and not learning to handle insulin reactions.

3. A sense of helplessness that blocks learning and action.

4. Unwillingness to ask for help from an informal support system.

5. Participation in a negative family or in social situations that detract from self-care.

If you feel you need more support than your network or group can give, take this as a sign of healthful perception, not as evidence that something else is wrong with you.

SETTING UP YOUR SUPPORT NETWORK

In some areas of the country, you can find an abundance of diabetes support activities. Local American Diabetes Association chapters, hospitals, clinics, or individual physicians may sponsor continuing support groups that you can attend. Your local ADA office should know if anything is available in your area. You may find that there are only general educational meetings. Although not specifically devoted to emotional support, these events are good places to meet other people with diabetes and their families and thus start building your diabetes network.

Cultivating this network—the informal cluster of people who share your interest in diabetes—is an effective and relatively easy way to develop your support system. You may find people who are already functioning as diabetes networkers, and they are often storehouses of information on people, resources, and meetings. "You're trying to get control of your eating? Talk to Joe Dodds. He's winning that battle and can really help you." "You're afraid of laser treatment and keep putting it off? Joan Mason can tell you how she overcame her fear." Don't feel that it is an imposition to ask for help. Most people genuinely enjoy an opportunity to help someone, especially when they share a condition as significant as diabetes. Networkers themselves are a special breed who love the process of making connections. As you gather information, you may find that you would like to serve in this way, too.

Talk to your friends and relatives, your druggist, your doctor and nurse, clinics or hospitals with diabetes education programs, and the nearest ADA chapter. Indicate that you want to get in touch with people with diabetes who have fairly positive attitudes and who could encourage you. If you need support, it doesn't help to begin networking with people who will make you feel worse.

You may run into some dead ends as you begin, so be prepared to persevere in building your network. Some doctors may feel very protective of you and may discourage you from learning from others with diabetes. And some people with diabetes avoid others like the plague. You may have to make a number of calls before you start getting positive responses, or you may find enthusiastic support right from the beginning.

Soon you will have several people you can call on when you need support or information. Perhaps there will be a person who shares a compulsive eating pattern with you, and you agree to call each other when the urge strikes. If you have a complication developing, you may want a buddy who has dealt with the same problem. Or you may just want a sympathetic ear when it all feels like too much.

Occasional telephone contact or conversation over a diet soda or cup of coffee may satisfy your need for support. You'll go through a sorting process, dropping out of contact with people who just complain and turn away from any encouragement. You may find friends of friends calling you because they have heard you are interested in mutual support.

You will soon be giving support to others, offering resources you know about: a new development in diabetes care you have just read about, a drugstore that sells insulin at a discount, a doctor who works well with patients. When you encourage another, you encourage yourself. A basic principle in mutual aid is that giving and receiving are really the same.

Sometimes you will be able to offer guidance or information well suited to someone else's needs. But there will be times when there is little you can do. Don't feel that you always have to have an answer. Your responsibility is to listen, to show that you care, and to share what you know. Sometimes "You'd better talk to your doctor about that" may be the most useful thing you can tell someone. As your network grows, you will also be able to suggest talking with other diabetics who can help with particular problems.

DEVELOPING A SUPPORT GROUP

Informal networking can provide very effective support, especially for people who are uncomfortable in groups. A regular group, though, offers certain bonuses. You can obtain feedback from a variety of points of view, and you have a larger body of experience to draw upon. A group can bring in guest speakers or even set up a training program in different aspects of diabetes management. People working together are usually more effective than individuals in handling the needs of members going through a crisis such as occurs when complications develop.

A support group is most effective when it is one activity of an ongoing network. If members feel free to contact each other between meetings, support is always available. Members maintain continuity of contact even though they may not be able to attend every meeting. The meetings themselves are more relaxed, since they are only one of several ways of sharing.

If you find no existing diabetes support group to join, you can start one by following the networking steps just described. Ask the people you contact if they are interested in helping to create the group. Find out what they are willing to do, what they want out of the meetings, and how often they would like to get together. You will find some who enjoy organizing and leading meetings, and others with practical skills like typing or access to copying machines. Assume that the work load will be shared and that you do not have to carry the whole burden. It helps to be clear about the tasks people take on and to specify when they need to be completed. "You're willing to call Sarah, Phil, Joan, and Larry? The meeting is on the tenth, so can you do that by the second?"

You may want to proceed informally, or you may prefer to set up a coordinating committee right at the beginning. Two or three other members are enough to work with you in organizing the group, planning meetings, and developing any other activities. It will become clear which decisions need to be made by the whole group and which by the committee. Some groups want to share in the organizational tasks and decisions, and others prefer to use most of their meeting time for support and learning. In your initial conversations with potential members, you will begin to get a sense of how they feel about this question. It can be explored at length in the first meeting.

The First Meeting

It is important to establish a positive tone at the first meeting, for without it, there may not be a second meeting. The details of this first meeting depend upon your style and that of the people you are working with. We will describe three alternative ways of conducting this session, but there are many others.

Alternative 1. Shared Leadership

Everyone shares in the creation of the group. At the beginning, the facilitator or discussion leaders ask the group to work together to develop guidelines, structure, and topics. Everyone in the group should answer the following questions:

- What do you want out of the group?

- What do you want to avoid?

- How do you want the group to operate—no leader, rotating leaders, professional facilitators?

- What guidelines for discussion are important to you?

- What are you willing to do to help the group function?

The leader encourages everyone present to describe his or her preferences. After discussion of each question, agreement may be reached, a vote may be taken, or further discussion may uncover solutions that satisfy conflicting views.

The strength of this approach is that it encourages a high level of participation and responsibility. In this way, it reflects the level of individual responsibility demanded by diabetes itself. However, if some group members are dealing with major problems, they may find it difficult to give their attention to discussion of organizational questions. If you know you have someone in crisis, find out—before the meeting—how they feel about this way of beginning the group.

There should be a definite cut-off point for the organizational discussion, and at least half of the meeting should be devoted to talking about living well with diabetes.

Alternative 2. Committee Leadership

A coordinating committee is responsible for defining initial guidelines and structure of leadership. This style may be appropriate if you sense that the people coming to the first meeting are on the shy side. The discussion leader briefly describes the proposed structure and asks for approval or recommendations for change. Then it is possible to move right into the support work. With good topics for initiating discussion, group members can quickly experience the value of being in a support group. But it may take more effort to involve them in keeping the group going.

Alternative 3. Outside Leadership

If you find that you or the potential members lack confidence in a self-directed group, a counselor or social worker might be hired to lead the first few meetings. You would need to look for someone experienced at facilitating groups and willing to build the group's capacity for functioning on its own. A local college, hospital, or public health department could help you find such a person, who might even be willing to volunteer the time. If not, the group would have to be willing to pay fifty to one hundred dollars for each meeting.

Any of these structures can be effective. Choose the one that feels most appropriate to the people in your group. For more information on conducting this first support meeting, see the general comments on meetings that follow, especially the sections on guidelines, stress level, and evaluation.

Conducting Successful Support Meetings

A clearly stated set of guidelines for meetings helps to instruct new members and remind old ones of the group's basic values and meeting style. The list can be printed or read at the beginning of the first few meetings. This helps to keep discussion within bounds and avoids pitfalls of discussing individual regimen in a group setting. Your group can create its own guidelines from scratch or use the following as a model.

Guidelines for a Diabetic Support Group

1. We are here to support each other in facing the challenge of living well with diabetes. By helping each other, we help ourselves. We intend to maintain a positive climate for discussing our experiences, feelings, problems, and solutions.

2. We will feel free to share any information about ourselves within the groups, but we will not disclose anything we hear to people outside the group.

3. We will respect each other's right to remain silent as much as his or her right to speak. And we will be sure to leave openings for the silent to speak.

4. The proper care of diabetes differs from person to person. We will remember that regimen is individual and not try to advise someone else on the basis of our own practice.

5. If we hear something that suggests possible changes in our own regimen of physical care, we agree to discuss such changes with our physician before acting.

6. If we feel anyone is passing on misinformation, we will not be afraid to challenge the information. When there is a difference of opinion or doubt, we will check out the facts with a health professional.

7. One of our functions is to share feelings. When we do this, we will give support but avoid interpretation and analysis. If any of us opens to deep emotions during the meeting, we will allow room for this. At the end of the meeting, one of us will check with the person to be sure he or she is all right.

8. We will feel free to express anger but not to direct it at other group members.

9. Many of the topics we discuss at an informational level may arouse strong feelings and stress reactions. When any of us senses stress

and tension growing, we will feel free to ask for a moment of silence to check our feelings. When the group stress level is high, we will take time for guided relaxation or another stress-reduction technique.

10. When one person is discussing a problem, we will encourage that person to find his or her own answers before offering ours. When we make suggestions, we will do it gently, without pushing.

11. If any of us is an alcoholic or a drug user, we agree to come to meetings only when we are sober or straight.

12. If any of us decides to stop coming because we can't handle the issues the group discusses or the way the group functions, we will discuss our reasons in the meetings or contact someone in the group and give feedback on what is causing the difficulty.

13. Having diabetes is a challenge to learn the lessons of life it brings to us. We are together to support this learning.

Leading Effective Meetings

These suggested guidelines imply that many of the leadership functions in a group can be shared by all the members. If each person takes responsibility for maintaining orderly discussion, awareness of stress levels, respect for feelings, and other questions of process, the meetings will practically run themselves. When there is clear understanding of the group's guidelines, it is even possible to function without a formal discussion leader.

However, it may be more effective to designate one person as facilitator or discussion leader for each meeting, with the role rotating to another member each time the group meets. This is especially true if new people come regularly.

The facilitator will do the following:

1. See that the group's guidelines are read at the beginning of each meeting.

2. Mention any departures from the guidelines if they occur.

3. Lead introductions and collect the subjects people wish to bring up.

4. Gently steer discussion, quieting side conversations and opening new subjects when the last has been completed.

5. Stay attentive to stress levels and call for relaxation when the level is high.

6. Reserve space for discussion of any group business, such as change in meeting place.

7. Conclude each meeting with a time of evaluation and appreciations.

When a different member handles this job at each meeting, the whole group becomes experienced in the skills required. It becomes natural for everyone to share the leader's tasks. Then, when the evening's facilitator fails to notice the high level of stress caused by a description of his or her own problems, for instance, anyone can call for a relaxation break.

Introductions

You can ask members to introduce themselves, describing their relationship to diabetes as well as saying something about their life outside diabetes. If they also mention any subjects they would like to discuss during the meeting, the evening's agenda is developed by the time they are finished. (The facilitator should list subjects, perhaps on a chalkboard or a large pad of paper.) Knowing who has type I or type II diabetes and who is a parent or spouse of a person with diabetes helps keep information relevant. The information about one's life outside diabetes helps group members see each other as complete persons, not just as people who have diabetes.

Starting Discussion

Reviewing the subjects people mention during introductions may be all that is needed to begin a flow of discussion that lasts all evening. The facilitator can read the list and ask the group which topic to take up first. Another way of beginning is to assign a subject that establishes a positive mood: "The most useful thing I've learned about living with diabetes is..." or "How has diabetes improved my life?" It is surprising how easily most people talk when such simple questions are presented.

Guiding Discussion

Sometimes meetings flow spontaneously, with little need for guidance from the facilitator. But there are times when some gentle steering is helpful. One person may be cut off prematurely. A quiet "I'm not sure Francis was finished speaking" will return the floor to the speaker.

There may be shy members in the group who will say little or nothing during the meetings. You can open space for them by saying, "Do any of the people who've not been saying much want to speak?" Allow them time to speak up, but do not pressure them. They may prefer to just listen for a while, and they will be able to learn from other people's experiences.

Setting a Positive Tone

A support group is more attractive if members emphasize abilities rather than disabilities, and solutions rather than problems.

Members need room for describing the difficulties they experience, but they should be encouraged to overcome these difficulties rather than be a victim to them. Pose questions in such a way that they elicit positive responses. Ask: "How do you deal with your feelings about diabetes?" instead of "What psychological problems does diabetes cause?"

Awareness of Stress and Feelings

Many of the things we need to discuss at a support group may raise the stress level for some or all of the people present. Feelings of vulnerability will be aroused by even the most boring and technical description of laser treatment: "My doctor shot this blue beam through a thick contact lens. The flashes were really bright. He said he did 800 zaps the first session." When the group is discussing highly charged subjects such as complications, it is important that the facilitator and group members watch for signs of rising stress. Some of these signs include a tendency to change subjects too quickly or to give in to nervous laughter.

It is always appropriate for any group member to ask, "Is anyone else feeling anxious?" and call for a stress check—a moment of silence in which people sense how they are reacting to the subject under discussion. If enough of the group shares the discomfort, the facilitator can lead a guided relaxation session. In this way, members learn to be aware of and manage stress as it occurs. This also makes participation in the group a more positive experience. A diabetes support group should reduce, not increase, the stress level.

Avoiding Misinformation

Members must feel free to challenge any information they believe to be inaccurate or incomplete. Keeping the facts straight is so important that a self-led group might enlist a physician or nurse practitioner to be a resource person who can be contacted by phone between meetings about questions that arise.

Handling "Difficult" Members

You may feel you lack the necessary assertiveness to confront the person who talks all the time, or the one who drains the group with chronic complaints and discouragement, or the one who sarcastically criticizes others. As facilitator, one thing you can do is refer the difficulty to the group as a whole: "Jim seems to have a lot to say tonight. Does anyone else want to say anything?" Or suggest doing something that will change the tone: "Betty has pointed out quite a few of the things she doesn't like about doctors. I'd like to hear if any of you have anything good to say about your doctor." Or just say what you are feeling: "I'm frustrated. It sounds like everyone's doing everything wrong, according to Cliff."

Evaluation

At the end of the meeting, each member describes what he or she most appreciated about the evening's discussion (and other members' contributions) and mentions any changes that would improve the sessions. This regular feedback helps keep the group on course.

Meeting Format

Support group meetings can follow a variety of formats. Each encourages a different style of discussion, so it is a good practice to vary the format occasionally. Some of the possibilities include the following:

1. General discussion following from the questions and concerns members bring up at the beginning of the meeting.

2. Sessions organized around a specific topic. The coordinating committee might choose the topic in advance, or the group could decide on one at the beginning of the meeting.

3. Discussion in subgroups: insulin dependent and noninsulin dependent; diabetics and nondiabetic family members; married and single people. With this format, people are able to spend more time on questions unique to being the spouse of a diabetic, a single diabetic, and so on.

4. Discussion in pairs. The group can break up into pairs occasionally, either to discuss an assigned topic or just to get better acquainted. This is an important variation for people who are more comfortable talking one-to-one than in groups. When the group reassembles, members may summarize their learning from the more intimate conversation.

5. Question-and-answer or instructional periods with a guest speaker. A nurse practitioner or psychologist might give instruction in stress management for diabetes. You might ask a physician to answer questions such as "How can we make the most effective use of our office visits?" A nutritionist might be asked to describe new research affecting diabetic diet. (Guest speakers can be effective early in the development of a group to enlist new members.)

6. Films related to diabetes as a way to focus discussion. *Diabetes— Focus on Feelings*, for instance, is an effective tool for a group exploring feelings about having diabetes.

7. Social events. Potlucks to share favorite dishes, parties, and picnics.

Some Topics for Discussion

- How has diabetes been my teacher, helping me learn about living?

- What attitudes, beliefs, or skills have helped me cope with diabetes?

- What do I wish I had known about living with diabetes at the beginning?

- What benefits do I receive from diabetes?

- What are three things I like most about myself? How do they (or how could they) help me deal with diabetes?

- What attitudes and skills do I need to learn to deal with diabetes better? How can I learn them?

- How does diabetes affect my relationships, both intimate and casual?

- How did I feel when I first learned I had diabetes?

- What can I do to create a more effective relationship with my doctor and health care team?

- Given my need to respect the demands of diabetes, what can I do to improve the quality of my life?

- How can we cut the costs of managing diabetes?

The elements you select for your diabetes support group and the ways you combine them are up to your particular group. There is no universal formula for support groups, just as there is no universal regimen for diabetes care. Feel free to experiment until you find the combination that works for all your members.

The following is a description of how one group met in Seattle.

A MEETING OF A DIABETIC SUPPORT GROUP

Five of the regulars are present at the agreed-upon meeting time, so they begin with guided relaxation and introduce the topics for the evening. Three more people, one of them new, come in during the introductions and join in. The newcomer says she wants to find out about blood glucose testing, so this is discussed first. The three members who are doing blood glucose testing talk about how it has improved their control. They recommend that the newcomer attend a class at a diabetes clinic. Later in the evening, the hostess brings out a blood test strip and a lancet, and the woman tests her blood, with participation of the others.

A man with type I diabetes and his wife arrive late because the man had a serious insulin reaction just before dinner. As he described what happened, it becomes evident that he is on a metabolic roller coaster. Group members emphasize the importance of working closely with one's doctor to get regulated. They also suggest some specific actions that would help: making his schedule more regular, keeping detailed records, handling stress more effectively, and sharpening his awareness of reaction cues. A young woman who has had diabetes most of her life says with conviction, "It is possible to learn to control diabetes."

The man's wife describes her distress over the difficulties she goes through with her husband. Others acknowledge that it can be as difficult to live with someone with diabetes as it is to be one. Another spouse offers to get together with the woman for coffee and share some of the things that have helped her live with her husband's diabetes.

One member notes that the stress level seems high after talking about personal relationships. She asks if others would enjoy a relaxation break. Many people nod, and the facilitator reads a guided relaxation exercise, going through the steps of the relaxation as she reads.

A 32-year-old woman works in an office says that she has been using the relaxation technique she learned at the previous meeting. She says she does it several times a day, and she believes that her blood sugar control has improved. She suggests relaxation to the man who had the reaction.

The facilitator notes that only thirty minutes of the meeting are left, and she asks how the group wants to end the meeting. The man who had been delayed by the reaction says he had been wondering if his difficulty with control had something to do with his beliefs. He asks people in the group to talk about the beliefs that help them maintain control. A thoughtful discussion follows in which people describe the beliefs that help them. The ones who feel they have very little control speculate on the beliefs they think might help them.

A coordinating committee member asks about the possibility of shifting the meeting to another night because of conflicts in several members' schedules. Another evening is found. Everyone agrees to meet on a different night next time. She also asks for a volunteer to type up a new membership list.

The meeting ends with the facilitator and other members expressing appreciation to individuals and to the group as a whole.

SUPPORT GROUP HOUSEKEEPING

Several practical aspects of an ongoing support group need to be handled. The two to four members of the coordinating committee can work with the group as a whole on these matters.

Information System

Coordinating committee members can be the ones who talk to potential new members and whose phone numbers are listed on any printed announcements. A membership list can serve as the basis for a phone chain that allows easy communication with the group between meetings. Each committee member calls two people, who each call two people, and so on through the list. The phone list indicates clearly who calls whom.

If the group wishes to grow larger, information can be distributed by networking through doctors, nurses, pharmacists, dietitians, friends, and relatives, as well as the local ADA chapter. If these channels fail to bring in the flocks, you can send press releases to neighborhood newspapers and make spot announcements on radio and television stations.

Group Size

This depends on space available and flexibility about meeting format. Large groups (more than ten members) can work effectively if they use subgroups and pairs fairly often to give everyone a chance to participate. Small groups can function well because of their close or personal nature.

Meeting Frequency

Every other week is probably the best schedule for the meetings. A weekly meeting may feel burdensome. Gathering once a month may not allow the group to develop momentum.

Meeting Place

Private homes, schools, churches, community centers, and bank meeting rooms are some potential meeting places. Some support groups meet in hospitals or public health buildings, but the association with illness may discourage some diabetics from coming. Using homes gives a more informal atmosphere. So long as the site is changed every month, meeting in homes does not become a burden on any one member.

Attendance

Some members may come regularly; others may drop in on the group only when they feel a special need. If the group is seen as only one function of a diabetes network, irregular attendance becomes less frustrating to the people organizing it. They can stay in touch with members by phone. People who do not appear regularly will know that they can always get support by calling or visiting another member.

Screening and Referring

Occasionally, a diabetic who clearly needs professional physical or psychological assistance may come to a support group. This might be someone who simply does not have a physician, someone dangerously out of control metabolically, or someone with serious mental problems. Only people who seriously disrupt meeting process should be screened out. But the group should not try to solve problems that call for skilled help. Members should clearly indicate that professional guidance is needed and, if necessary, help the person find a physician or mental health professional.

OTHER ACTIVITIES OF THE SUPPORT NETWORK

Many other support activities can be initiated by your diabetes network. Your network may or may not be related to the local chapter of the American Diabetes Association. Some chapters are fairly conservative and diabetics may find an independent organization more creative than working through the official group. The power of your network can be directed to opening such chapters to more input from diabetics. If your local ADA already has a good level of partici- pation, any of the following activities might be easily accepted.

Training for Support Giving

Diabetics and family members can learn communication skills, stress management, problem-solving techniques, and guidelines as to the limits of peer support. Such a training program might be developed with the aid of mental health professionals from a local college or community clinic. (Crisis clinics often have volunteer training work- shops that could be adapted to the needs of diabetics.)

Support for New Diabetics or Diabetics in Crisis

Beginning with visits to new diabetics still in the hospitals after diagnosis, or at home if the person has not been hospitalized, network members can provide desperately needed encouragement and practi- cal information to patients and their families. They can also visit people in the hospital after a major emergency such as diabetic coma, insulin reaction, or treatment for complications. This is a time when one's motivation to improve self-care is high. Contact with a fellow diabetic who has gone through similar crises and learned from them can be inspiring. Many ADA chapters have a special program for newly diagnosed diabetics.

Study Groups

People who are interested in learning about a particular subject might form a study group. For instance, three or four people interested in learning the intensive regimen might work together, helping each other master information they need to attain optimal control. This would make the learning process easier and ensure the emotional support needed to make such basic life-style changes. Or people with retinopathy could work together collecting and sharing information on the condition and its treatment.

Residential Houses

A live-in treatment center for adolescent diabetics was operated in Gainesville, Florida. This was available for children who had serious difficulties managing diabetes. The program included individual and family psychotherapy and intensive instruction in diabetes care. When families were willing to participate in the center activities, the children showed a significant improvement in management. A diabetes network could take the lead in developing professional and community support for the creation of such a center.

SUMMARY

We can draw powerful support from the community of people who have diabetes—the people who best understand the meaning of living with diabetes. We can work together to deal with feelings, to share information, and to learn the new skills needed for diabetic management. This can happen individually, through personal networking, or in support groups that meet regularly. Both styles of giving and receiving support are effective. If diabetes networks or groups do not exist in your area, you can create them using the information in this chapter.

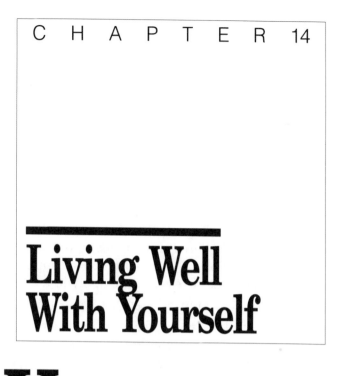

C H A P T E R 14

Living Well
With Yourself

You are one of the best available sources of support for living well with diabetes. You are always there. You know yourself well. No one else can take care of you as well as you can.

The way you feel about yourself affects your willingness to live healthfully. And having diabetes can affect how you feel about yourself. The goal of this chapter is to help you become aware of the personal strengths and resources within you and to learn how to neutralize patterns that weaken your ability to care for yourself well.

You are resourceful. You are stronger, more creative, and more able than you usually realize. Some of these strengths may be hidden, some may be used in only one corner of your life, some may be expressed in negative ways. All your strength can be redirected to increase your ability to live well with diabetes.

For example, the teenager who refuses to test or to follow diet or schedule is showing great strength of character. This strength is focused on rebellion and denial, but it is a valuable resource. This teen can learn to turn "won't power" into "will power" and improve his or her self-care.

After months of receiving support, a man acts the weak and pathetic victim of diabetic complications. He is overwhelmed, helpless, and depressed. Where is his strength now? Perhaps he is very strong in the tenacity with which he holds onto his role as victim, refusing to adapt to his situation. Feeling sorry for oneself consistently takes enormous energy. The self-image of weakness can be recycled into the true flexibility that a person needs to live well with the changes being experienced. The source of many negative feelings can be redirected into positive action. This redefinition of apparent flaws reveals a surprising new set of resources to apply in a healthy way.

Often you develop skills in one realm that you never use in the rest of your life. Photographers, for instance, learns about tests, measurements, precision, and combining a complex series of actions to achieve a given result. They clearly have the basic skills needed for learning a diabetic regimen. Salespeople are skilled at communication and persuasion. Perhaps they could use these strengths to sell themselves an improved regimen.

Let's explore the store of resources you can use to live well with diabetes.

GOING INTO YOUR STOREHOUSE

Do this exercise in a quiet place where you won't be disturbed. At each step, close your eyes and allow both words and images to come to mind to help you find answers. Then make notes before you go to the next step.

1. Think of any three areas of your life, large or small, in which you are successful. See yourself in action. What strengths do you demonstrate here?

2. Think of three activities you truly enjoy. See yourself enjoying them. What personal qualities do you have that allow you to enjoy these activities?

3. What do you believe about yourself that enables you to act with success? With enjoyment?

4. Remember one of the best times in your life. Tell yourself the story of that time or recall scenes from it. What qualities of yours made this such a good time?

5. What strengths do you draw on in your work (or schoolwork, if you are a student)?

6. What personal strengths do you express in your relationships with friends?

7. What special qualities do you experience only when you are alone?

8. If you were to fulfill your true potential, what hidden qualities would you feel free to express?

9. What qualities would you like to develop?

10. What are some of your most negative traits or limitations?

11. Can you find a strength that each of these limitations contains? Can you think of a way to turn it to serve you?

12. Now, review your answers and examine how these qualities can:

   • Help you deal with diabetes.

   • Enable you to improve your physical self-care.

   • Help you feel better about having diabetes.

   • Assist when you are fearful or unwilling to do what you know you should do.

   • Allow you to resolve problems in relationships with others.

Write down your thoughts or discuss them with a friend.

In the days after you first do this exercise, observe your life with these questions in mind. See what other traits you can find that could help you live well with diabetes. Continue exploring how the qualities you have just identified could improve your self-care.

Recognizing your inner resources will help you feel you have the power to deal with diabetes creatively. You can support this positive step by learning to overcome whatever negative self-image, limiting beliefs, self-judgments, emotional reactions, and behavioral patterns you experience because of diabetes.

A CASE OF MISTAKEN IDENTITY

Beliefs, feelings, and actions work together in a system that forms your sense of who you are. You tend to become closely identified with this system, forgetting that it is only a set of patterns you learned. Many of your limitations seem so real and deeply rooted that you can't imagine being anything more. You forget that you *learned* to see yourself as inadequate or helpless or rebellious or sick.

This mistaken identity become self-perpetuating. When you believe you are weak and unable to follow your regimen, you act weak and unable. Then you may feel depressed and eat a pint of ice cream. Now even your sugar-clogged body feels uncomfortable. The evidence grows. Beliefs, feelings, and actions interact to reinforce each other and strengthen your negative self-image.

Responses to the threat of diabetic complications illustrate the way false identity functions as a circular system of beliefs, feelings and actions.

If you believe that diabetic complications and an early death are inevitable, you are likely to feel anxious and fearful or possibly depressed. Or you may bury your feelings and live for the moment, hurrying needlessly or ignoring the actions that could improve your odds. The idea creates the feeling. The idea and the feeling together lead to action. When you believe nothing will do any good, you may do little or nothing to manage your diabetes. Or, with great anxiety, you may manage so compulsively that your stress level decreases the benefits of a tighter regimen.

On the other hand, if you believe you can reduce the risk of complications and early death, you become more hopeful. Anxiety may still be with you, but you learn to handle it and return to positive feelings. When you do, it is much easier to follow your regimen and do the things that reduce your risks. Following your regimen encourages positive feelings, and the immediate benefits support the belief that it does make a difference.

In both cases, beliefs affect feelings, beliefs and feelings affect actions, and the actions then affect the beliefs and feelings. Neither pattern is an inevitable response to having diabetes. Either way, consciously or unconsciously, you choose the way you respond. You can choose to become aware of any of your beliefs, feelings, and actions relating to diabetes and to change them when they lead to negative results.

Change comes from seeking a deeper identity and detaching from seeing ourselves as our limitations. Not, "I am weak, sick, and unable," but, rather "I am the person who can see these negative patterns without judgment. I am the person who chooses the life I live. I am the person who learns, who grows, and who changes. With this image of myself, I find it easier to use the strengths implicit in all I have learned."

With this self-image as a foundation, you can work for specific change at the level of belief, feeling, or behavior, whichever suits your style best. Or you may move from one level to another, integrating changes in beliefs, emotions, and actions.

CHANGING BELIEFS

A belief is a statement about yourself or about the world that shapes your life. It may be conscious or unconscious. Some beliefs give you power; some make you feel weak.

> I am capable of learning to manage diabetes; or
> I just can't manage; it's all too complex.

> Diabetes is a teacher, challenging me to be my best; or
> Having diabetes is a punishment.

> People accept me as I am; or
> People judge me for having diabetes and think I'm a bother.

Some beliefs are limiting, restricting your ability to act and producing feelings of helplessness. Others are enabling, giving more power and encouraging positive feelings. The limiting beliefs are often so deeply ingrained that you believe them to be absolutely true. They tend to be reinforced by the feelings and actions that result from them.

If you believe you cannot control the amount you eat, your actions keep proving you to be correct. Then you feel depressed and eat even more to bury your feelings. Such vicious cycles can be broken by recognizing that beliefs like these are not truths but only learned habits of thinking. When you view them as mental habits rather than facts, you begin to reduce the power they have over you.

Of course, many of your beliefs will be related to factual knowledge. It is a fact that people with diabetes have a higher risk of kidney failure than the general population. It is a mistake to build on this fact the belief: "I will have kidney failure." A more appropriate belief is "I can act to reduce my risk of kidney failure." This one gives you power and also has a factual basis, because most diabetics do not develop kidney disease.

UNCOVERING YOUR BELIEFS ABOUT YOU AND DIABETES

Watch for hidden beliefs as you work on diabetes learning, especially at times when you feel stuck. Catalog the major beliefs that both empower you and limit you in your life with diabetes.

Some techniques for uncovering beliefs are as follows:

1. Ask yourself a repeating question: "What do I believe about _____ (diabetes, home blood testing, complications, my diabetic regimen, how diabetes affects my relationships, my doctor, my old age, etc.)?"

    Another way of doing this is to alternate between "What do I believe about _____?" and "What should I believe about _____?"

    Repeat the question for each topic a dozen or so times, writing down whatever beliefs come to mind.

    Example: What do I believe about myself as a diabetic?

    Sample — *Beliefs:* I am more vulnerable than other people. I should get special consideration. I will probably die in my sixties. My problems are a bother to others. I am unwilling to follow a strict regimen; this is a sign of weakness. Others should take care of me. I really want to be fully responsible for myself. I have learned to live better because of diabetes. I value my life because I know how vulnerable I am.

2. In a concrete situation—especially at a time of distress, frustration or failure—ask "What beliefs have created this problem?"

    Example: I have "forgotten" to take my morning dose of insulin and don't notice the signs of high blood sugar until late afternoon. (I am scheduled for a job interview that day.)

    Sample — *Beliefs:* If I'm sick, I won't be held responsible for anything. Diabetes isn't really serious. I'm invulnerable. Hurting my body is better than facing difficult challenges. I'm weak and deserve to be hurt. I want someone to take care of me.

3. Choose an enabling belief you would like to adopt. Calmly repeat it, holding out one hand as though it were speaking the belief. Let the other hand state the limiting beliefs that oppose it. Keep repeating until you understand the conflicting beliefs and the conflict starts to dissolve.

    Example: Right hand: A blood sugar test is free of judgments.
    Left hand: It shows I've eaten like a pig.
    Right: A blood sugar test is free of judgments.
    Left: Big Brother is watching me.
    Right: A blood sugar test is free of judgments.
    Left: It just makes me worry to see how high the test can be.
    Right: A blood sugar test is free of judgments.
    Left: Can I ever learn to control myself?
    Right: A blood sugar test is free of judgments.
    Left: I'd like to stop worrying so much.
    Right: A blood sugar test is free of judgments.
    Left: I really want to know the truth.

4. Write or speak a fantasy in which you are easily doing something that now feels difficult or impossible. Write down all the reasons the fantasy could not come true. Then write down the beliefs that would enable you to make the fantasy real.

After completing any of these exercises, underline the beliefs that seem most powerful, indicating the ones that limit you and the ones that free you. Then choose the limiting ones you would like to change.

Bringing limiting beliefs into the open is a first step toward changing them. Sometimes the new awareness itself is enough to dissolve the power a belief has over your feelings or behavior. Or you may have to take further steps to replace the belief with one that enables you to live as you wish.

There are many techniques for changing beliefs. Some are developed by behavioral psychologists, others by people in the human potential movement. (Techniques 3 and 4 in the preceding section are good for changing as well as uncovering beliefs.) A few techniques for changing beliefs are as follows:

1. Create a positive phrase in present tense that clearly states the belief you want to adopt. Use your own words. Find ways of reminding yourself that this new belief is entering your life (for example, put signs around the house and repeat the phrase with feeling every day).

   Example: To replace the phrase "I am unable to follow diabetic regimen" try "I am improving my regimen step by step. I am able to continue until I have excellent control." The new belief is encouraging but not overwhelming.

2. Relax and imagine yourself doing the specific things that would indicate you are living according to the new belief. Let a concrete scene unfold in your mind where you see (or feel) yourself acting as you wish to.

   Example: With "I am improving my regimen..." I see myself testing blood, keeping records, rejecting extra food, exercising, and doing the other things that mean improvement for me.

3. Recycle scenes from your life in which a powerful limiting belief was active. Recall the scene in detail, noting how the belief was expressed in your feelings and actions. Then imagine how you would have lived the scene if you had held the new belief at that time.

   Example: My old belief is "I must keep my diabetes a secret. I'll be rejected if people know."

I'm embarrassed at lunch because a friend keeps insisting I eat her cake and I don't want to tell her I have diabetes. I'm afraid she won't go out with me if she knows. I get angry and uptight. She is hurt.

I want to adopt the new belief "I am open about having diabetes. Anyone who rejects me isn't worth having around anyway."

I see myself at lunch, smiling when my friend presses me to eat the cake. I say, "I've got a little secret I'm going to let you in on. I'd love to eat the cake but I really can't. I have diabetes." I sigh as she responds with surprise and caring. I answer her questions without embarrassment and feel deeply relieved to have torn down that wall between us.

4. Trace the roots of beliefs and cut them. You learn your beliefs. The strongest ones you learn from your parents or other people who have had a parental influence. When you have trouble weakening a particular belief, it helps to determine who you learned it from. You can even see yourself giving it back to the source, or cutting the connection. With a belief specific to diabetes, you may have to look for a generic idea underneath it.

    Example: I have a set of related beliefs: "I am more vulnerable than other people. I should get special consideration. I will probably die in my sixties." These beliefs are clearly from my father, who had rheumatic fever as a child. He was sure he had cancer years before it finally developed. He was 67 when he died.

    I would rather believe: "I am both vulnerable and strong. I will give myself special consideration by living well. I will die when I die, and I can't predict when that will be."

    I see myself telling my father why I won't follow his example anymore. I give him a box containing his old beliefs and he throws it into the fire. He smiles at me and says, "Go ahead. You are free to outlive me."

    Beliefs are closely related to emotions. Working at the level of beliefs can help relieve negative feelings. And it helps to have tools for working directly at the emotional level.

DEALING WITH FEELINGS

Living with a complex, life-threatening condition like diabetes adds many emotional triggers to our lives. The threat of long-term complications creates an underlying anxiety for many of us. A delayed meal, a cut foot, or having no sweets available when blood sugar swoops low can become major emergencies. Diabetes even affects our relationships with others.

Our feelings have very direct effects on diabetic control through the stress response and through their effect on our willingness to follow our regimen.

Throughout the book, we have examined a number of the emotional issues specific to diabetes. We focus here on ways of gaining awareness of and handling your feelings as they relate to your self-care.

The following exercises will help you sharpen your emotional awareness and capacity for more effectively working with your feelings.

In this work, you may find strong emotions coming to the surface (particularly if you are in the midst of dealing with a tough situation). If you are not used to feeling things very deeply, this can be an alarming experience. You may want the aid of a friend, support group, or professional.

What am I feeling?

1. Breathe. A very simple way of finding out what you are feeling is to sit quietly and breathe a bit more deeply than usual. Feel your stomach, your chest, your throat, and your face. Relax and breathe and allow the feelings to emerge.

2. Imagine. Visualize in whatever sense you use (sight, sound, body movement, smell, or taste) to form images of what you are feeling. Let scenes unfold in your mind that act out your feelings.

3. Move. Let your body tell you what you're feeling by moving or dancing. Allow the movements to come spontaneously, without worrying about appearing graceful.

4. Descend. Often there are layers of feeling below the emotion you're conscious of, all crying to come into awareness. The experience of being stuck in a feeling may stem from the deeper feelings underneath it. Breathing, relaxing, and visualizing are ways to sink into these deeper layers. After you've experienced each level, ask yourself, "What feeling is below this one?" Then sink down, as though going through the floor.

(The exercises for getting in touch with beliefs in the previous section are also likely to bring feelings to the surface.)

Just getting in touch with an emotion often will be all you need to do about it. You feel it for a time, you may express it, and then go on with life. At other times, a feeling may seem eternal and inescapable. Perhaps you've just seen a diabetic relative who has recently become blind, and you feel down for a week. You've been on a food binge for two days and are filled with guilt and anger at yourself. You can probably supply your own examples all too well.

What you can do about feelings

1. **Accept what you are feeling and experience it.** Don't compound the problem by chastising yourself for feeling the way you do. You have every right to feel whatever you are feeling. Use the techniques described above to explore this experience with a sense of curiosity.

2. **Express the feeling.** With the mode of expression that feels most appropriate, communicate the emotion that you feel stuck in. Draw or paint, write poems, speak to a friend (or into a recorder), sing or dance. Communication often enables you to let go of a feeling that seems endless.

3. **Detach from the feeling.** Detachment is not suppression of emotion. It is a refocusing of awareness to a broader sense of yourself. The emotion is there, along with the detailed experience of your bodily sensations, your perceptions of the world around you, and a center of awareness that observes your feeling, sensing, and perceiving.

Example: I am feeling hopeless. Depressed. Dark. I can't escape this feeling. I sense my feet on the rug, the texture of the rug. My breath is shallow. My nose is dry as I breathe. I want to escape, go to sleep. I've never felt such deep despair. I see wind blowing trees outside the window. I hear the wind in the leaves. My stomach is tight. I smell the rose across the room. I hear music from downstairs. It's a song I like. My chest relaxes when I think of the words. Depression seems like a ball inside of me instead of me locked inside it. The ball is dissolving. My breath is deep now. I have tears in my eyes. I'm alive again.

"It should recompense us well to study the qualities of our emotional spectrum, studying them not as a pathologist dissects but as an artist cares for his materials. Or perhaps as one who loves. For the quality of our emotions belongs to ourselves perhaps more than any other aspect of being. To love ourselves, then, means to love these pure qualities. In a strange way purely expressed emotions engender a degree of empathy and love as part of our interrelations. 'Seeing' them as they are eases the burden and boundary that separates man from man."

—Dr. Manfred Clynes

Changing behavior

Discussion of the third area of change important to living well with diabetes, how we act, extends throughout this book. The introduction and Chapter 1 in particular explore the techniques and attitudes that support changing our behavior. Rather than repeating any of these themes we ask you to review the introduction.

TELLING THE STORY OF YOURSELF

Earlier in this chapter, we emphasized the interaction between the three levels of life: beliefs, feelings and behavior. Now we would like to explore the integration of the three. Work on any one of the levels produces change, and at some point you will want to bring them all together. This may be after you've gained greater clarity or it may be when you are feeling so stuck you don't know what else to do.

A powerful way of integrating levels is to simply tell your story.

See your whole situation by telling yourself what is happening. Move back and forth between what you are feeling, the beliefs and mental images that surround your feeling, and the things you are doing. See how the different levels reinforce each other. Identify the specific limiting beliefs that have gotten you stuck, if that's where you are. Recognize how your actions feed the feeling and demonstrate the truth of the beliefs.

You can write this narrative or say it aloud to a friend or into a tape recorder. Use the most direct language you can.

> *Example:* I'm frustrated, angry and guilty. I've been on a binge for two days and can't stop. I have no self-control. I'm probably taking years off my life when I do this. I must hate myself. I started eating Tuesday morning, just after Dr. Blast told me my tests were lousy and that I really had to take better care of myself or I'd be in for real trouble. I've been trying so damned hard and it just doesn't do any good. Nothing I do works out right. Why can't he understand how hard I've been trying?
>
> Now I'm poisoning myself with candy and pastries. My blood sugar must be 500! Every time I eat something I feel worse. I'm angry at how weak I am. Afraid I'll never learn how to take care of myself. Afraid of what this is doing to me.
>
> Oh! There's a blind woman at the newsstand in the lobby of Dr. Blast's building. I never even noticed her before Tuesday. I forgot about her right away, but now I can see her face so clearly. I'm terrified I'll go blind like her. I don't believe there's anything I can do. I can't do anything right.
>
> No wonder I'm in such a pit. I must be stronger than I think if I can keep myself feeling this bad and acting so stupid for so long. My eyes are still fine. There's still lots I can do to keep them that way. Dr. Blast was worried and doesn't know how to be gentle. I can be gentle. Gentle and strong.

This example focuses on a specific situation. You can also gain great insight by telling your story in a more expansive fashion. Describing your life with diabetes through the years can give you extraordinary perspective, balance, and understanding. You might do this with a friend who has diabetes or another medical condition, swapping stories at length.

When you have reached a point of achievement, narrating the tale of how you got there both rewards and reinforces the changes you have made. You need not be bashful about giving yourself credit for the work of living well with diabetes.

Living well with yourself is, finally, a matter of balance—balance between the needs of diabetes and the other demands in your life; and balance between acceptance and reaching out for something better. As this sense of equilibrium grows, you will find that it endures as a deep source of inner support, even in times of turbulence and upset.

Section V
LIVING WELL WITH DIABETIC COMPLICATIONS

CHAPTER 15

Neutralizing The Threat Of Complications

"Complications?! I don't want to hear about them. That's too depressing."*

If that's the way you're feeling when you turn to this section, we can sympathize. After living with diabetes for about forty years each, your authors have experienced all the fears and uncertainties you may feel. One of us, Ernest, has experienced a major complication—temporary loss of vision in one eye and then when that cleared, a temporary loss of vision in the other. Treatment was successful, and Ernest's vision is still clear nine years later. So we know there is hope to counterbalance the threats implicit in this subject.

Absorb the challenging information contained in the next three chapters, and you will have the ability to improve your odds for avoiding complications. You may limit, postpone, or even avoid altogether the effects of diabetic complications on your future health. You will know what you can do to increase your chances of preventing them. You will know what their early warning signs are so you can seek treatment in time. If you are already dealing with their unwelcome arrival, you will have tools to avoid their dominating your life, no matter what disabilities they bring.

Complications are not an inevitable process in diabetes. How we live with diabetes can slow and even reverse the development of its side effects. So make a date with these chapters—today, tomorrow, next week, next month, whenever you're ready, but soon!

Roget's Thesaurus comes close to capturing the emotional quality of the word complication when it gives *entanglement, snag, snarl,* and *difficulty* as synonyms. Diabetes by itself is a relatively friendly condition. But when we consider its potential complications, it can become intensely threatening.

An essential part of the diabetes self-care package is staying open to new information about this topic we love to avoid. Face the fears that it brings up, and go ahead and face the facts. This doesn't mean studying every last detail of what can go wrong, but you do need to know the following:

• Changes in regimen and life style that will reduce your risk.

• Early warning signs that enable you to seek prompt treatment if a complication starts to develop (both laboratory test results and signs that you can recognize yourself).

• Treatments now available and under research for each complication.

• Ways of reducing anxiety over the possibility of developing diabetic complications or dealing with feelings that come up if they do begin.

• When you know these things, you have the power to turn the odds in your favor. You may be able to avoid complications altogether, or if they do develop, escape their more serious consequences.

In these three chapters:

• We examine recent developments in diabetes care that can reduce the risk of complications emerging.

• We offer attitudes and techniques for dealing with the anxiety, fear, and uncertainty engendered by the threat of major complications.

• We explore the physical and emotional needs of the person who is experiencing the onset of a major complication of diabetes.

• We discuss the specific long-term complications of diabetes and the steps you can take to improve your chance of escaping them.

290

Taking It Easy

No other aspect of diabetes education is as promising—or as threatening—as the subject of diabetic complications. We want you to live well while you work with these chapters. That means taking it easy, pausing, relaxing, using other techniques for reducing stress, and remembering that the very act of reducing stress is likely to reduce your risk of developing complications. Our purpose is to convey the idea that you can do many things to reduce this risk, not to overwhelm you with the risk itself.

Special care must be taken in discussing complications with diabetic children.

NEUTRALIZING THE THREAT

We are at risk for serious disabilities and early death, yet we can live well with the risks and the anxiety they evoke. What could better express the central concept of this book? We can reduce both the risk and the anxiety. Even if we are disabled by one or more complications, we can still go on living well.

We have said many times that diabetes is a teacher. Here the lessons are powerful: living peacefully with physical and emotional risk; accepting vulnerability while living a full life; coming to terms with aging and mortality; identifying with inner healthfulness, no matter what the state of your body. When you deal with the questions raised by complications, you can't help but grow as a human being.

A medical dictionary defines complication as a disease process that may or may not accompany a primary disease. Possibly you have had a doctor who warned you of your higher risk of stroke or heart attack. Or you may have diabetic friends or relatives who have become blind or whose kidneys have failed. You may have read of the diabetic nerve disorders that can result in loss of feeling, in pain, or in impotence.

The possibility of developing these complications is the most serious consequence of diabetes, so serious that many of us avoid facing it. (Avoidance has been reinforced by the tendency of some parents and doctors to use the threat of complications as a motivation-through-fear device.)

"I ignored my fear of complications. I felt good so I didn't give them a thought. I knew that complications existed for other people—but not for me. Then all of a sudden I was realizing, I'm a little lazier, more lethargic. I feel drained. It gradually got worse, to the point of my kidneys failing."

—Jim

We feel that hope is a much better motivator than fear. You have a solid new basis for hope—you can limit or avoid the effects of complications. To do this you need to be informed, and you need to find that willingness to act on what you learn.

Three Anxiety-Reducing Ideas Concerning Complications

1. Complications are not inevitable. You have a risk but, fortunately, no guarantee that you will develop major complications of diabetes.

2. You can reduce your level of risk by improving your diabetes self-care program, maintaining better control of blood sugar and blood pressure, practicing stress management, and exercising regularly.

3. Treatment for most complications is becoming more and more effective. In many cases, their negative results can be reversed or reduced, especially when detected early enough.

These three ideas provide an essential context for considering diabetic complications, so we will examine them here in detail.

Complications are not inevitable

When you read statistical reports on diabetic complications, you may believe you cannot escape them. "Blindness is 25 times more common in individuals with type I diabetes" is a typical statement. Those are dramatic odds, but actually, less than 1 percent of us loses our vision. The majority of people with diabetes do not become blind. Even without doing anything special, you have a good chance of escaping a major handicap.

Statistics are misleading—if not terrifying—for a very fundamental reason: They are based on an earlier era of diabetes care when the medical knowledge and tools we have now were not available. It was a time when individuals were much less interested in a healthy lifestyle. Some important research questions are still unanswered, but the statistics for the present generation of diabetics will be improved.

Michael and Cousin Melvin

Ernest counseled a 13-year-old boy named Michael who had developed diabetes six months earlier. Michael's doctor had asked him to test his blood sugar, but he seldom did so. "It reminds me of being in the hospital at the beginning. They were testing me all the time," Michael complained. Ernest asked what the tests had meant to Michael. "They remind me I'm diabetic. I want to forget it. I don't care." Michael talked more about being in the hospital. "I kept hearing about my uncles and how they died of diabetes when they were in their forties."

"Michael, I think it's time you heard about my cousin Melvin. He became diabetic the year after they first used insulin with people. He's almost 80 now and he's still going strong. No complications most of that time. What happened to your uncles doesn't happen to all of us!"

Ernest asked Michael if he'd like to adopt a cousin. Melvin agreed to this, and the next week Michael said he'd told everyone about his new cousin Melvin. He wanted them to know he had a chance.

You can reduce your risk by improving your management of diabetes

You can tip the odds in your favor by the way you live. Older studies of people maintaining a moderate level of control showed they were less likely to develop major complications. Now that a near-normal level of control is possible, you can reduce your risk even more. The risk is still there, but it is much smaller. Diet, exercise, blood pressure control, and stress management also make complications less likely to occur.

(The development of complications is determined by a number of factors other than metabolic control. Inheritance, stress, and other matters of life-style may also play significant roles in any particular case. So it is possible to be well controlled and still experience a serious impairment.)

Treatment for most complications is becoming more effective

If a complication does develop, you are more and more likely to find a treatment that will reverse or limit its advance. This is especially true if you are aware of early warning signs and seek treatment promptly. Thousands of diabetics are escaping disability thanks to laser treatment, kidney transplantation, early treatment of foot disorders, and other new developments.

But There Are No Guarantees

In spite of all these advances, real risks are still present for you. There are many variables: how long you have had diabetes, at what age it began, the kind of lifestyle you have had, your genetic makeup, and other individual factors still poorly understood. You can do everything possible to reduce your risks of developing complications, and they may still occur.

So diabetes makes a clear demand: Learn to do your best and at the same time live well with uncertainty. Learn to cope with anxiety and return to hope, no matter what happens. This is not too different from the demand the world at large makes upon us all.

You and Diabetic Complications

This exercise will help you see how you relate to the possibility of diabetic complications developing. Answer spontaneously, even though the feeling or belief that comes may seem "wrong."

1. What did you feel as you read the beginning of this chapter?

   _____

   _____

2. Which of the following statements describe(s) the way you have dealt with complications in the past?

   ——I don't want to think about the possibility of complications.

_____I worry about them quite a bit.

_____It makes me angry that diabetes could do that to me.

_____I do everything I can to reduce the risk.

_____I could do more to reduce the risk.

_____I just do everything I want to, since I don't know how long I'll last.

_____I probably spend too much time taking care of my diabetes.

_____I feel depressed quite a bit.

_____I feel guilty because I have not taken good care of myself.

3. I believe I will probably live to the age of _____

4. The complication I fear the most is _____

5. I tend to believe

_____I will escape major complications.

_____I will certainly develop a major complication.

_____There is nothing I can do to change what will happen.

_____If one complication develops, others will surely follow.

_____If I become (or am) disabled in any way, my life will be damaged beyond repair.

_____I will be able to learn to live well with the disability.

_____I will be a burden on others.

Other beliefs I hold about complications include _____

Positive beliefs that would neutralize any negative beliefs listed above include _____

6. Is there anyone close to you who keeps reminding you of what can go wrong? Who uses threats to motivate you? Have any of your doctors done this?

7. My present level of control is_____. My level of regimen is _____ (See your questionnaire results in Chapter 4.)

8. I intend to make the following improvements in self-care in the next months _____

9. I can get support for my feelings about complications and for making changes from _____

10. I do not intend to make any changes in self-care at this time because

    _____I am already doing everything possible.

    _____I do not believe it would do any good.

    _____I do not feel I have the time and energy needed.

    _____I feel the changes would reduce my freedom or pleasure.

    _____I feel overwhelmed by the demands of diabetes.

    _____Other_____

    _____If someone you loved gave the reason(s) checked above for not improving his or her care of diabetes, what would you say to that person?_____

Make an appointment with yourself to reopen this question in a few months. Mark it on your calendar.

Reflect on your answers to these questions. Look for changes in beliefs or behavior that will help you to lessen the threat of complications. For example, if you do not feel you have the time and energy needed to improve your self-care program, ask yourself what changes in your life would give you that time.

DEALING WITH ANXIETY ABOUT COMPLICATIONS

Undoubtedly the best way to deal with anxiety about diabetic complications is to do as much as possible to reduce your risk of developing them. A complete diabetic regimen makes complications less likely at the same time that it handles your day-to-day need for metabolic control. The following list indicates the things you can do.

WAYS YOU CAN REDUCE YOUR RISKS

1. Improve your metabolic control and continue improving it to the best level you are comfortable with.

2. Learn to handle stress well.

3. Follow a diabetic diet that features low fat and high fiber, as well as limitations sweets and rapidly absorbed carbohydrates.

4. Exercise regularly.

5. If you are overweight, lose weight.

6. Act to prevent high blood pressure by controlling stress and weight. Seek treatment for hypertension if your blood pressure is high (above 140/90).

7. If you smoke, quit.

8. Get the amount of sleep and rest that you need.

9. Know the warning signs for each complication.

10. Consider taking a multivitamin pill even though there is no compelling evidence that this will do more good than a balanced diet.

Except for item 1, this is the same prescription for good health doctors give nondiabetics. It is especially important for you because each item on it will improve your odds of avoiding other disease as well as escaping diabetic complications (or of limiting them if they have already started).

You may have already adopted some of the measures and need to make only a few changes. Or you may need to alter your life in every area. Begin where you feel most willing to change; or, if your sense of urgency is great, begin with metabolic control, the most fundamental way of reducing risk. You give yourself the best chance for a long and healthful life by following the complete preventive program as soon as you can. At least give yourself the benefit of some stress reduction and self-acceptance if you choose nothing else from this list. Only you can define the ingredients of a life-style that will work for you.

More on Reducing Anxiety

Assuming that you are doing everything on the preceding list or are in the process of learning to, you may still experience anxiety. So one of the useful skills to develop is the art of living well with uncertainty. For all the talk of risks and odds and possibilities, you simply cannot know if you will or will not end up with one or more diabetic complications. You can do your best to avoid them, and then a special sort of surrender to uncertainty is necessary. You squarely face the possibility that you will become disabled as a consequence of diabetes. And with equal power, you face the possibility that you will remain free of major complications. You decide you will live well with yourself, no matter which path is given to you. And you return to the immediate task of living well right now.

Learning about complications should be a gentle process in which you use stress-reduction techniques to their fullest: relaxation, meditation, prayer, and whatever else is effective for you. Take in information in small doses, and give yourself intermissions that allow you to focus on positive, optimistic aspects of life. Participation in a diabetes support group or one-to-one conversations with other diabetics can help you deal with the feelings that come up. Some diabetics will find a few counseling sessions helpful while they are dealing with this threatening subject.

Another way of dealing with your feelings at this point is to explore the beliefs and attitudes you have about the possible consequences of diabetes. Neutralizing crippling beliefs and adopting more positive ones can help relieve the anxiety, depression, or anger that you may experience. For instance, a typical belief is, "I've been so out of control that I can't possibly escape complications." In any individual case, this is a belief, not a fact. A more useful belief to replace it is, "If I improve control now, I may still escape major complications."

IF YOU DECIDE NOT TO ACT NOW TO REDUCE THE RISKS OF COMPLICATIONS

You may feel unwilling at this time to make the changes in your life that would lessen the risk of complications. If so, it is vitally important that you make this a conscious choice. Look at the reasons you give for maintaining your present level of self-care. Discuss them with someone you trust. Explore them fully within yourself, through writing, inner dialogue, prayer, meditation, or whatever means works for you.

See if you can find a new point of view that allows you to begin making the necessary changes while still dealing with whatever is valid in your reasons for not changing. For example, if lack of time is your main reason for not changing, find changes that do not require additional time, or learn to use your time more effectively.

And, if you consciously choose not to change, accept your decision and any anxiety that goes along with it. You are increasing a set of risks in your life, but you are not guaranteeing the development of complications. We all make risk/benefit decisions about our lives each day. Self-acceptance is itself healthful for body and mind. And it gives you a positive foundation for making new decisions in the future.

We suggest you make a date with yourself a few months in the future to reopen the question of what you are then willing to do to reduce the risk of complications. Your life may or may not have changed enough that other choices are available.

If Complications Develop

"**H**ow long can you mope and pine after disaster? You've got to ultimately pick up your life and sing."

Rev. Karl Baehr
(Diabetes Forecast, *Nov./Dec. 1983*)

"When my kidneys started to go, it stimulated me to educate myself. I put time and energy into finding out what I could do to help myself. It was a great deal of motivation. It scared me a lot. I knew how sick I could become. That terrified me—what my body could do with me having no control over it. I also realized there was something I could do to gain control."

—James

THE EARLY SIGNS

Usually diabetic complications show early signs of development. They may appear in laboratory tests, you may notice the signs yourself, or your doctor may notice them during a routine exam. Your ophthalmologist may tell you that you have background retinopathy, a condition found in the majority of people who have had diabetes for ten years or longer. Or your physician may tell you the beginning signs of kidney disease are present, shown by protein in your urine.

You may shrug off the diagnosis, or you may find the news very disturbing. But this "bad news" can provide the motivation you may need to improve your regimen dramatically. Action now may enable you to delay or halt the progress of the disorder, and perhaps even reverse it. (The early signs of each complication are described in the next chapter. If you know these warning signals, you will be able to avoid delay in beginning preventive treatment.)

THE CRISIS BEGINS

The onset of a major diabetic complication is a crisis, no matter how well you handle it. It reminds you of your vulnerability. The beginning of one disorder may suggest that others will follow. You may feel angry and frustrated if excellent self-care has not prevented complications. At the same time such feelings come up, you may have to make serious decisions about treatment and changes in life-style.

All of this adds up to a major life challenge that demands your time and energy and the support of others. You will live well through this crisis if you deal with the many practical, emotional, and social needs it generates.

At first, however, you may react to the crisis in a way that allows you to deal with the shock of diagnosis. Some people go through a stage of denying that anything is happening and try to ignore both the doctor's recommendations and their own feelings. Others enter a period of withdrawal and defeat while they absorb the impact of the news. Still others become convinced that the worst will happen to them. Some feel guilty. Others go on a food binge, believing that nothing does any good anyway.

Understand what your own pattern of response to diagnosis of a complication has been. If your response is negative, do not fault yourself for reacting in this way. You had to deal with a stressful piece of news. But recognize the limitations of this initial reaction and allow yourself to move on to a more functional response.

Treatment and Self-Care

You may have to absorb new information quickly, learn new skills, make important decisions, and change some basic elements of your life at this time. These changes may feel overwhelming, especially when you are still trying to deal with your feelings. You can regain control of the situation if you clearly define the tasks facing you. Break them down into manageable steps. Establish how much time is needed, what resources and support you must line up, and what information you must acquire. By organizing the demands, you tame them. (The questionnaire at the end of this chapter will help guide you through this process.)

You will probably be faced with decisions about treatment and regimen. In some cases, specialists may describe fairly complicated procedures that would be difficult to follow even if you were not under emotional stress. If you do not understand what is being recommended, say so, and ask for explanations in language you do understand. If you still don't understand, ask your internist or family practitioner to help you. Ask if there are written materials or audiovisual aids describing the treatment. You have a right to understand fully what you are being asked to undergo.

You should know what the risks of the recommended treatment are. What are the odds for success? For a negative outcome? What is likely to happen if you do nothing? Are any alternative treatments available? If you have any significant doubt about the course of treatment your doctor suggests, seek a second opinion from another physician with equivalent expertise. (For instance, do not go to a general practitioner or an internist for a second opinion about eye treatment. You need an ophthalmologist, preferably one who specializes in retinal diseases or even diabetic retinopathy.) If your doctor does not have much experience working with diabetes, you probably should find someone who does to guide treatment of the complications.

In addition to prescribing a specific treatment, your doctor may suggest that you improve your regimen of self-care at this time. Improvement in blood sugar control may help you handle the condition that has developed. It may also make other complications less likely to occur. You will need to *proceed cautiously in tightening metabolic control if you have advanced retinopathy or kidney disease.* In a number of studies, these complications worsened (at least initially) when good control was gained too quickly. When retinopathy (at the proliferative stage) or kidney disease is clinically evident, blood sugar levels must be lowered gradually, over a period of three or six months. This is true whether control is improved through multiple insulin injections or the insulin pump.

You may need to be cautious in your exercise and physical activity at this time, depending upon the specific complication you have. This is especially true if you are starting an exercise program after years of relative inactivity. You should discuss exercise and physical activity with your doctor. You may want to enroll in a medically supervised exercise program that monitors your physical condition.

This may also be a good time to improve your diet. You can begin by eating more fresh vegetables and fruits and cutting down on animal and saturated fats. You could add more beans, pasta, and other high-fiber foods to your meals.

Coping with the Emotional Impact of Complications

Having a diabetic complications is inherently stressful, so this is an especially important time to manage stress well. Stress from any source interferes with your control of blood sugar, and it plays a role in the development of diabetic complications. Do your best to limit other sources of stress in your life. Learn to relax under anxiety.

The emotional impact of the changes in your body is a highly individual matter. You may feel overwhelmed, or you may come out swinging. You may feel frightened or depressed or angry. You may do your best not to feel anything at all. If a major body function is involved (loss of vision, amputation, or kidney failure), it is natural to go through a grieving process. In any case, you are likely to find yourself going through a series of emotional reactions, rather than experiencing just one. Allow yourself to feel what you are feeling, but if you become stuck or find that you are unable to act, ask for help.

Family and friends may be able to assist. Or a support group, guidance from others who have gone through what you are facing, or professional counseling may be required. This is a time when most people need some form of support. Immediate family members usually experience their own stress about what is happening to you, so it is best not to rely solely on them. (In some cases, their input may be so negative that it is better to seek all support elsewhere.) Other diabetics who have weathered the storm will know what you are going through. They may be able to help you sort things out at a practical level and offer encouragement at the same time. If informal support is not enough, you may want to see a psychotherapist (psychologist or psychiatrist) or a social worker who specializes in medical counseling.

The onset of a diabetic complication is a time when you may gain a new appreciation of your own internal resources for coping. Such a crisis often puts you in touch with your greatest personal strengths and spirituality. You may gain encouragement from remembering the resources that helped you through difficult times in the past. Chapter 14, "Living Well with Yourself," describes many techniques to help you handle your emotional responses at this critical time.

IF COMPLICATIONS DEVELOP

The diagnosis of a diabetic complication is a major life challenge. This questionnaire will help you clarify what is happening, how you are responding, and what you need to do.

1. What diabetic complication(s) has your doctor diagnosed?_____

    _____

2. At what stage of development is the complication?_____

    _____

3. What treatment does your doctor recommend?_____

    _____

4. What risks are involved with this treatment?_____

    _____

5. What are the odds for a successful outcome? _____

    _____

6. What does your doctor think will happen if you do nothing?_____
   _____

7. What changes in regimen or life style does your doctor suggest?__
   _____

8. Do you think you will have any trouble making these changes? (If so, go to Chapter 3, "Help!")_____
   _____

9. Outline the individual steps you need to take to make these changes. Also include any decisions you need to make about treatment or things you have to do to undergo treatment. _____
   _____
   _____

10. How are you coping with the diagnosis of the complication so far?

    ____I am trying to ignore what the doctor told me.

    ____I am ignoring my feelings.

    ____I am paying attention to my feelings.

    ____I am reading everything I can get my hands on about the complication.

    ____I am talking with people who have been through this.

    ____I am feeling withdrawn. I don't want to talk to anyone.

    ____I am worrying a lot and dwelling on the worst possible outcome.

    ____I am blaming myself and feeling guilty.

    ____I am living it up. I'll enjoy myself while I can.

    ____I am doing everything possible to take care of myself.

    ____I am becoming too dependent on my family or friends.

    ____I feel absolutely overwhelmed.

    ____Other_____

11. How would you like to change your reaction?_____

12. How are you feeling about the diagnosis?

    _____ Angry

    _____ Frightened or anxious

    _____ Guilty

    _____ Depressed

    _____ Hopeless

    _____ Hopeful

    _____ Grief-stricken

    _____ Calm

    _____ Other_____

13. What support can you count on? (Name the people.)

    Family_____

    Friends_____

    Diabetes network_____

    Other support network_____

    Professional and religious counselors_____

    Other_____

14. If you do not now have enough support, what steps can you take to find the help you need?_____

FOR YOUR FAMILY OR FRIENDS...

Someone close to you is going through a crisis, and, most likely, you are too. Give him or her all the support and encouragement you can, and seek the same from others for yourself. This is a time when you will all be drawing on inner resources, and, with luck, becoming closer.

If at first, you find your loved one (or yourself) reacting negatively, understand that something shocking has occurred. If the negative reaction in your loved one persists, gently suggest some appropriate responses. If your own reactions remain negative, seek outside help for yourself and try to find others who can give support to your friend until you can.

Find a balance in the assistance you give. Issues of dependency may arise. Your friend may feel he or she is being a burden or may attempt to be overly independent. Help define where help is and is not needed. Don't reinforce feelings of inadequacy by doing things he or she would rather take care of. But also be realistic about any physical limits imposed by the disorder.

Complications Simplified

> **"I** *want to know the risks I'm facing as a dia-
> betic. Why stick my head in the sand and
> pretend I'm not worried? I tried that and it
> didn't work worth a damn. I kept hearing horror stories, anyway. I
> finally pushed through my fears and read about all the things that
> could happen to me. Glad I did. I found out what I could do to improve
> my odds for avoiding them."*
>
> *—Marybeth, 50 years old*
> *Forty years diabetic with only minor complications*

In this chapter we review background information on the causes of
diabetic complications and the possibility of reversing or preventing
them. We also offer a comprehensive program for reducing your risks
of developing complications. We review in detail the nature of the
major disorders of diabetes, specific preventive measures, and the
options for treatment.

If you feel tempted to skip this chapter, we suggest you read at least
the sections describing what you can do to avoid the various complications. This is the most important reading you can do. Then, later,
return to read the rest of the chapter.

WHY DO DIABETIC COMPLICATIONS DEVELOP?

Although medical library shelves bulge with studies trying to answer this question, it still is not fully resolved. Still, the broad outlines of an answer do exist.

One major explanation centers on the many abnormalities found in the system of a person with poorly controlled diabetes. The basic inner ecology is profoundly out of balance, especially in the circulatory and hormonal systems. When blood sugar is chronically high, excess sugar disrupts the structure and biochemical processes within the body's cells, particularly those of blood vessels, nerves, kidneys, and eyes. These repeated imbalances create the building blocks for diabetic complications. There is increasing evidence that some of these building blocks are the result of excess glucose reacting with protein in the body, creating AGEs (advanced glycosylation end products). For example, a recent study showed that AGEs accumulate faster in the arteries and circulatory system in diabetic patients than nondiabetic patients. The increase was positively related to the severity of diabetic kidney disease in these patients.

One imbalance caused by high blood sugar is hormonal. When combined with the biological disruption of emotional or physical stress, the damage from this is compounded. This means that stress management can play a vital role in reducing your risk of complications.

One crucial result of circulatory changes in a tendency for diabetics to develop high blood pressure. Though hypertension has no symptoms of its own, it contributes strongly to the development or worsening of retinopathy, kidney disease, and cardiovascular disease. If hypertension is present, control of blood pressure may be as important in preventing complications as keeping blood sugar levels down. (The life-style factors associated with high blood pressure include obesity, high intake of salt, smoking, stress, and lack of exercise.)

Finally, recent studies show increasing evidence of the importance of genetic factors in complications. We inherit tendencies toward or resistances to some of the disorders related to diabetes.

310

So, in any individual case, the onset of a diabetic complication will be determined by a unique combination of past blood sugar imbalances, hormonal imbalances, hypertension, environmental influences, and genetic tendencies.

CAN COMPLICATIONS BE PREVENTED OR REVERSED?

This question has been a subject of medical controversy that is only beginning to be resolved. Some diabetic nerve disorders have been reversed through stricter control. Retinal disorders have shown mixed results, with improvements in some cases. Kidney disease in diabetes may be influenced more by high blood pressure than by high blood sugar.

While the evidence is still fragmentary, many researchers believe that tight blood sugar control can prevent or reverse some complications and delay the onset of others. But major questions remain unanswered: How early must one maintain this level of control in the course of diabetes? How do the different factors that cause complications interact? How do other aspects of self-care influence the risks? Are the benefits worth the costs in time and effort and risks of acute insulin reactions?

Diabetes research examines relationships among a limited number of factors—control of blood sugar levels and development of complications studied statistically in a group of people. But the situation of each of us as an individual is influenced by a whole life system generally outside the researcher's capacity for study. Diabetic control must be seen as one of a variety of factors determining our future—diet, exercise and activity level, patterns of managing stress, emotional life, immunological responses, heredity, and other influences yet to be discovered.

If we look at the question of preventing complications in this broader frame of reference, improving blood sugar control becomes one important part of a healthy, balanced life-style that is of immediate and long-term benefit to people with diabetes. In the face of researchers' specific uncertainties, the total benefits of improving diabetic control are well worth the costs. The degree of control you maintain, though, must be

311

determined by your other life demands and the need to avoid acute insulin reactions. That is why we describe three levels of control to help in your decision making. Our goal is to help you be realistic in your choices and not fool yourself about what you are and are not willing to do to control your diabetes.

Diabetes Control and Complications Trial

A study of over 1,400 people with diabetes will bring more understanding to some of these issues as results begin to be reported in 1994. (Early reports have already begun.)

The ten-year study is being conducted to determine the effect of strict blood sugar control: Can it control, prevent, delay, lessen, or reverse diabetic complications? What level of control is needed? What are the consequences—costs, benefits, side effects—of such tight control?

There is already a great deal of evidence on this question, generally suggesting that strict control reduces the risk; but many details still need to be studied.

REDUCING YOUR RISK OF DEVELOPING COMPLICATIONS

If you believe the hoped-for cure for diabetes or breakthroughs in treatments of complications will allow you to forget about preventive measures, don't fall for this illusion. The building blocks for diabetes' side effects accumulate over time, cause deterioration of basic body systems, and, in many cases, are not reversible. If you just wait for discovery of the cure, it may not work for you because too much damage may have already occurred. Preventive measures, started as early as possible, are much more effective than later treatment.

We will expand upon the list of actions you can take to reduce the risk of complications that appears in Chapter 15. "Reducing the risk" does not necessarily mean "avoiding complications." This is not always possible. But by following these preventive measures, you will improve your odds. If complications develop, they are likely to appear later, progress more slowly, and be more treatable, perhaps with methods not yet perfected or discovered. It is also likely that there will be fewer of them to deal with.

Ways to Reduce Your Risk

1. Improve your metabolic control and continue improving it until you achieve the best level with which you can live well.

    While other factors play important roles, blood sugar control is clearly central to reducing your risk for diabetic complications.

    Improvements in your level of control will make complications less likely to develop or delay their onset and severity. As we have said before, there is no guarantee, simply improved odds.

2. Learn to handle stress well.

    In the short run, poorly managed stress interferes with blood sugar control, causing either high tests or swings between high and low. In the long run, excessive levels of stress hormones are probably a major contributor to many diabetic complications.

3. Follow a diet low in fat, high in fiber, and with controlled salt consumption, as well as limitation of sweets and rapidly absorbed carbohydrates.

    Low salt consumption helps control high blood pressure. Restrictions of cholesterol and total fat, especially animal fat (and other saturated fats like coconut and palm oils) helps maintain a healthy circulatory system. In addition to having a beneficial effect on blood sugar, high-fiber diets have been associated with a lower incidence of colon diseases, including cancer.

4. Live an active life style and/or exercise regularly.

    Exercise provides a foundation for good metabolic control as well as helping control weight and stress. It also has significant benefits for cardiorespiratory fitness.

5. If you are overweight, lose weight.

    In addition to contributing to metabolic control, weight loss will decrease your risk for cardiovascular disease and hypertension.

6. Act to prevent high blood pressure by controlling stress and weight. Seek treatment if your blood pressure is high (above 140/90).

High blood pressure dramatically increases the risk of kidney failure and visual loss from retinopathy. As in people who do not have diabetes, it increases the risk of heart and circulatory illness. A program of prevention and treatment can be found in the section on hypertension later in this chapter. Following this program is one of the most important preventive actions you can take.

7. If you smoke, quit.

Smoking usually increases the risk of vascular disorders and heart disease, risks already heightened in diabetes. Smoking has a negative effect on arteries, small blood vessels, blood pressure, and circulation, thus contributing to arteriosclerosis, hypertension, and coronary artery disease.

8. Get the amount of sleep and rest that you need.

Adequate sleep and rest minimizes stress and contributes to good metabolic control.

9. Consider taking a daily multivitamin.

Scientific evidence supporting the preventive role of vitamin and mineral supplementation in diabetes is sketchy. Many claims for substances such as vitamins E and C, bioflavonoids, and brewer's yeast are made in health magazines, yet few reliable studies support these claims. There may be definite benefits in moderate vitamin and mineral supplementation. The medical community is more actively studying these substances in general, as well as for their particular use in people with diabetes (e.g. the value of the anit-oxidant properties of certain vitamins, and the possible benefits of magnesium or chromium supplements in certain people with diabetes.

Large doses of vitamins C (thousands of units per day) and E (over 250 units per day) should be avoided if advanced retinal disorders (proliferative retinopathy) or kidney disease (nephropathy) have developed. Such megavitamin self-treatment may have a damaging impact on these conditions, increasing capillary fragility.

This is not an all-or-nothing program. Each item on the list improves your chances. If you want to do more than you are now doing but have difficulty making all of the changes suggested, review the information on learning and change in Chapter 1.

THE MAJOR COMPLICATIONS OF DIABETES

The following catalog describes the conditions specific to diabetes or that take a special form in people with diabetes. We have not covered the cardiovascular complications whose course is similar in those with and without diabetes. You can find good sources of information on heart disease at the end of the chapter.

As you read this part of *Living Well,* be aware of the stress it is likely to trigger. Don't just plow through it, ignoring the feelings that naturally arise as you study such threatening material. Pause often, relax, and reassure yourself. Talk about your feelings with someone close to you, or write them down. Live well, even with this very difficult information about diabetes.

Complications of the Eyes

Diabetic Retinopathy

What Goes Wrong?

Abnormalities in blood sugar level, blood chemistry, and hormone levels produce an oxygen or circulatory shortage in the eye's retina and blockages of small blood vessels. At first, this results in background retinopathy—minor changes in blood vessels of the retina. When the process intensifies, new blood vessels form in the retina in an attempt to increase the supply of blood and oxygen. These vessels are weak and prone to leak blood and fluid into the retinal tissue or the vitreous liquid (the jelly-like substance between the retina and the lens) of the eye. Together with other blood vessel abnormalities in the retina, these hemorrhages can lead to decreased or total loss of vision. These changes also create a risk of retinal detachment or macular edema (excess fluid in the portion of the retina used for sharp vision).

Signs and Stages of Development

Background retinopathy begins to develop after five to twenty years of diabetes. It is a mild condition characterized by small, scattered changes in the retina. Vision is not affected, and the disorder is no cause for the alarm. The condition can be detected only through an ophthalmological examination by a doctor trained to recognize it.

Proliferative retinopathy may develop after fifteen years of diabetes, but it may develop sooner. New fragile blood vessels and fibrous scarring are found on the retina. Unless there is retinal detachment or hemorrhages interfering with vision, it can only be discovered through an eye examination. (Possible visual cues of this condition include the presence of flashing lights, floaters, and blurred vision.) Photos of your retinas may be taken, with and without a fluoroscein dye, to indicate points of leakage.

If proliferative retinopathy continues to develop, vision-blocking hemorrhages or retinal detachment may occur.

Macular edema is a thickening of the retina or the collection of fluid around the central part of the retina used for fine vision (the macula). This thickening results in blurring or fuzziness of vision.

The Risk

More than 90 percent of type I patients have mild or background retinopathy after fifteen years of diabetes. By twenty years, 50 percent have developed some degree of proliferative retinopathy. Before laser treatment was introduced, many patients experienced severe visual loss or blindness from advanced retinopathy. This risk has been dramatically reduced by the laser. Relatively few now become blind from this condition. For patients with type II diabetes, proliferative retinopathy is less common—after twenty years only about 20 percent of insulin-users and 10 percent of non-users develop proliferative retinopathy.

Prevention

1. Have an ophthalmologist examine your eyes each year after you have had diabetes for five years. Even if your vision is normal, you may have changes that can benefit from laser treatment.

2. Check your own vision *in each eye* weekly (or even daily), looking for any changes: increased blurriness, floaters, fuzzy areas. (Good vision in one eye may mask worsening vision in the other, so make sure you close each eye to check the sight in the other.)

3. Report any changes in vision to your doctor immediately.

4. Keep blood sugar as close to normal as possible.

5. Maintain normal blood pressure. (Practice preventive measures for high blood pressure.) Adhere to treatment for hypertension, if prescribed.

6. Maintain normal weight.

7. Avoid smoking.

Treatment

Your internist or family physician is trained to examine your eyes for retinopathy, but after five years of diabetes, you should have a yearly examination by an ophthalmologist. All treatments for retinopathy are performed by ophthalmologists. Once the first stages of proliferative retinopathy are diagnosed, you may need examinations every three or four months.

Laser photocoagulation is the recommended treatment for retinopathy once a certain level of new vessel formation or macular edema is reached. This is an office procedure in which an ophthalmologist uses a laser to make hundreds of microscopic scars along the retina. A local anesthetic can be used, but usually the process causes only moderate discomfort. The treatment increases the oxygen available to the central area of the retina and promotes healing of the new vessel growth. This decreases the risk of blindness by 50 to 60 percent.

Risks of treatment, occurring very rarely, include further bleeding and inadvertent scarring of the central area of the retina.

Possible side effects include a moderate restriction of peripheral (side) vision, a slight decrease in sharpness of vision, and decreased night vision.

A large, multi-center national study (the Early Treatment Diabetic Retinopathy Study, ETDRS) has shown that "focal" laser treatment decreased visual loss by about 50 percent in those patients with clinically significant macular edema. This is defined very precisely for the ophthalmologist and requires a special, painless exam. You may have clinically significant macular edema that would benefit from treatment, but you may not know it because your eyesight is still normal. *It is essential that you have your eyes checked even if your sight appears unaffected.*

Vitrectomy is a surgical procedure used when retinopathy is too far advanced to be treated by laser (because extensive hemorrhages fill the vitreous fluid in the eye, blocking the retina). The fluid is removed and replaced with a clear saline solution. The operation may also remove scar tissue and fibers that can cause retinal detachment. This process is riskier than laser treatment, so ophthalmologists usually prefer to wait six to twelve months to see if blood in the vitreous will clear without treatment.

Cautions

If proliferative retinopathy has developed, you should avoid activities that cause a sudden rise in blood pressure or a sudden flow of blood to the head: straining with bowel movements, bending over quickly, high diving, scuba diving, lifting heavy weights, head stands, and so on. Hemorrhages in the eye can result from these activities as well as from blows to the head. Discuss the general level of physical activity appropriate for you with your ophthalmologist.

At the proliferative stage, you should not tighten control quickly. Control should be improved gradually, over a period of several months. A sudden change to tight control can cause retinopathy to worsen at this stage.

It is important to cope with the emotional stress accompanying this threat to your vision. High levels of stress can add to the threat through the periods of high blood pressure they may cause.

Chronic high blood pressure should be controlled with medication.

High doses of vitamin C (over 500 mg per day), used by some to treat colds, should be avoided. This vitamin in large doses affects blood clotting and thickness.

Diabetic Cataract

What goes wrong?

The lens of the eye becomes cloudy as an indirect result of high blood sugar. The immediate cause is an excess of sorbitol, the alcohol of glucose, in the lens. This changes the chemical balance of the lens because it tends to accumulate in the cells. (Diabetics may also be more likely to develop the more common age-related form of cataract.)

Signs and stages of development

Cataracts affect vision differently, depending upon the pattern of cloudiness that develops in the lens. Opacity may occur at the center, around the sides, or diffusely throughout the lens. The initial stage of development may be detectable only through ophthalmological examination. In the mature phase, a milkiness can be seen from the outside, and vision decreases, with fogginess and halos around lights.

Prevention

1. Maintain excellent blood sugar control.

2. Some biochemical research indicates that taking 1,000 mg of bioflavinoids daily may help. This food supplement may reduce sorbitol in body tissues.

3. Research is now being conducted on aldose reductase inhibitors, drugs such as sorbinil, which counter the action of the enzyme that converts sugars into the sorbitol causing cataracts. If successful, a drug may be available to prevent diabetic cataract formation.

319

Treatment

Cataract surgery involves the removal of the cloudy lens, replacing it with a plastic lens. This process is usually done under local anesthesia. It restores vision in 90 to 95 percent of patients. Surgery is really indicated only when the disruption of vision interferes with your daily life.

Risks

This procedure incurs the usual surgical risks of infection and bleeding that can further compromise vision. The risk is low.

Take a Break

Especially if you are reading straight through this chapter, you need one. Relax, check your feelings, and give yourself some warm love and friendship. Taking in all this information is a difficult task. Do not imagine that you can just absorb it without emotional impact. After working with these hard facts for years, your authors still feel them deeply.

Kidney Disease (Diabetic Nephropathy)

What goes wrong?

The kidney filters blood, clearing out waste products and recirculating blood chemicals and proteins that are then reused. This is achieved by networks of capillaries (called the glomeruli), fine blood vessels that can become severely damaged by years of high blood sugar. A layer of the capillary—the basement membrane—becomes thickened.

With this thickening, kidney function is progressively altered. The selective filtering by the kidney is impaired. First, protein (albumin) that should be retained in the bloodstream is passed through the kidney into urine (a condition called microalbuminuria and albuminuria or proteinuria). Then, toxic waste products that should be filtered out of the blood remain in circulation (azotemia). Serum creatinine and BUN (blood urea nitrogen) levels become abnormally increased. (Creatinine and BUN are chemicals normally found in the blood and passed into the urine. Their levels rise if the kidney is not working well. Temporary increases may occur occasionally from causes such as eating a large quantity of meat.)

This stage eventually leads to a condition known as uremia: an excess of urea and other nitrogen wastes in the blood that produces symptoms of kidney failure, such as fatigue, decreased appetite, nausea, and vomiting.

The good news is that for patients who have had diabetes for more than forty years and have not developed proteinuria, it is unlikely that nephropathy will develop. Moreover, it appears that 60 to 70 percent of patients with insulin-dependent diabetes will never develop clinical kidney disease.

Signs and stages of development

The early stages of kidney disease are revealed only by urine and blood tests. We provide technical information on these signs to help you understand the results of tests your physician may report. The early signs of kidney disease can be strong motivators for preventive action on your part.

Stage 1

Changes in the kidneys begin to develop slowly over many years, with no obvious clinical signs or symptoms. The normal kidney excretes a small amount of protein (albumin) in the urine (less than 30 mg in a 24-hour period). With new, more sensitive tests, it is now possible to measure such small amounts clinically (rather than in a research lab). A urine protein level between 30 and 300 mg per day is called microalbuminuria.

Substantial evidence now indicates that persistent microalbuminuria predicts the later development of diabetic kidney disease (particularly in patients with insulin-dependent diabetes). So urine protein in this range—30 to 300 mg per day—along with the typically increased blood flow and filtration rate through the kidneys, can now be considered Stage 1. If nephropathy is going to develop, this stage may last an average of fifteen to seventeen years and has traditionally been considered the silent period of nephropathy.

Stage 2

The next development may occur after fifteen to seventeen years of diabetes on average. Standard urine tests may show abnormally increased albumin excretion, greater than 250-300 mg per day. At this stage, the kidney is leaking out protein, but BUN and creatinine— other indicators of disease detected through blood tests—have not yet started to rise. If Stage 2 is reached, development of further disease is highly likely. Proteinuria may be present in urine for several years without other evidence of kidney disease. (Remember, there is great individual variation for these statistics, and many diabetics never develop kidney disease.)

Stage 3

In this stage, BUN and serum creatinine levels slowly begin to rise. Once an individual's creatinine exceeds 2 mg/dl (milligrams per deciliter), it is possible to estimate roughly the time progression of disease and the percentage of kidney function remaining. Divide the creatinine level into 1 and multiply by 100 to get the percentage remaining. For example, a creatinine level of 4 gives approximately 25 percent remaining function. (Most patients don't have symptoms until function drops to 5-15 percent.) Your physician can give you a rough estimate of the rate of progress of kidney disease.

Stage 4

At this point, the kidneys are failing. BUN and creatinine levels have risen high enough that symptoms of kidney failure are occurring. These symptoms include poor appetite, vomiting, ankle swelling or other signs of fluid accumulation, weakness, lethargy, drowsiness, fatigue, and nausea. Weight gain, mostly from excess fluid accumulation, is continuing to occur. Do not scare yourself with the presence of any of these symptoms. Individually they are signs of a large variety of low-threat disorders. Laboratory urine and blood tests interpreted by your physician are the only way to determine the presence of kidney disease.

In Stage 4 kidney disease, dialysis or kidney transplant is necessary to preserve life.

Monitoring and Prevention

Although no evidence suggests that improved blood glucose control will affect the course of disease progression once Stage 2 has begun, there is some initial evidence that action in Stage 1 may benefit you. Researchers recommend that you generally strive for control as good as possible when your tests show microalbuminuria (30-300 mg/dl).

The following guidelines for monitoring kidney function are one approach:

In the first five years of diabetes, you should have a routine check for protein in the urine each time you visit your physician and a test for microalbuminuria at least yearly. BUN and creatinine should be measured at least yearly if proteinuria is present, and creatinine clearance every two years.

After five years or in the postpubertal patient, in addition to the above, you should have a 24-hour urine test yearly to measure total daily protein.

Once overt (dipstick) proteinuria or elevated serum creatinine or BUN is detected, kidney function should be monitored at least two or three times a year. Consultation with a nephrologist (kidney specialist) is necessary to plot a long-term therapeutic strategy and to discuss the possibility and implications of renal failure with the patient.

Additional preventive measures in kidney disease

1. Maintain the best possible metabolic control.

2. Avoid ketoacidosis (diabetic coma) by careful management of infections and stress.

3. Avoid high blood pressure through weight control and limited intake of salt or sodium (i.e., no added salt). Adhere to any hypertension medication prescribed. (Hypertension promotes the development of diabetic kidney disease.) Some antihypertensive drugs like ACE inhibitors or certain calcium-channel blockers may be especially useful for people with diabetes.

4. Use relaxation techniques as a further way of lowering blood pressure.

5. Avoid urinary tract infections. (Know the symptoms: burning or pain on urination and cloudy urine.) Seek treatment promptly if they occur. Such infections can contribute to kidney damage.

6. To minimize the risk of infection, you should not be catheterized unless it is absolutely necessary.

7. Use of dye-contrast agents in X-ray or other radiological studies should be avoided unless absolutely necessary. (They tend to be toxic to the kidney.)

Treatment

In the first stage, your internist or family practitioner is equipped to watch for signs of advancing kidney disease. By Stage 2, a kidney specialist (nephrologist) should be consulted to monitor your condition. Treatment in Stages 3 and 4 is by a nephrologist, preferably one experienced in diabetic kidney disease.

Stage 1

Strict adherence to preventive measures described above is likely to allow you to avoid or postpone diabetic kidney disease. The fact that you have an early warning sign in the microalbuminuria test gives you a valuable gift of motivation. The best possible self-care can keep your kidneys intact.

Stage 2

With excellent self-care—including all the preventive measures just described—you can probably extend the life of your kidneys by many years. Blood sugar control, weight control, and treatment for high blood pressure and urinary tract infections are the key ingredients of treatment here. Care at this stage is designed to extend kidney function by controlling hypertension and avoiding urinary tract infection and drugs toxic to the kidney (such as those used in some radiographic studies).

Stage 3

At this stage, your kidney function has deteriorated and toxic products are building up in the bloodstream. Blood sugar control may help other body systems but it cannot reverse kidney disease at this stage. Dietary restriction of protein may be recommended, although this is still an area of controversy. More specialists are recommending high protein intake (especially animal protein) even in Stages 1 or 2. Diuretic pills to help you lose any accumulated fluid may be prescribed.

Stage 4

Once kidney failure occurs, the two choices for treatment are dialysis or a kidney transplant.

Dialysis is a demanding procedure in which a machine performs the blood-filtering function of the kidneys. You are attached to the machine, using blood vessels in your arm, typically for four hours, three times a week. The experience is taxing, but it can add years to your life. Peritoneal dialysis uses the peritoneum (the lining of the abdominal cavity) to filter toxins out of the blood. It is possible to do this procedure at home or at work, and it may provide a motivated patient with more flexibility.

Kidney transplants allow a more normal life than dialysis. The technique is advancing rapidly, increasing the acceptance rate and long-term survival rate. Successful transplantation no longer depends on your having a kidney from a relative, since matching of cadaver kidneys has improved significantly. Five-year success rates range from 70 to 80 percent, depending upon the source of the kidney donated.

Cautions

Avoid ketoacidosis (diabetic coma), urinary tract infections, use of dye contrast agents in X-ray studies, and catheterization; follow treatment for high blood pressure.

Time for Another Break

Even if your kidneys are still completely healthy, what you have just read may be frightening and depressing. If you actually have signs of kidney disease developing, you will probably need to deal with strong emotional reactions. Chapters 3, 11, and 14 can help you handle these reactions. Don't be afraid to seek outside aid in a diabetes or kidney disease support group or from professionals.

Nerve Disorders (Diabetic Neuropathies)

What goes wrong?

Several families of nerve disorders may develop as complications of diabetes, producing pain, lack of sensation, digestive and urinary difficulties, and impotence. Fortunately, many of the disorders usually disappear after a few months to a year. Others are successfully treated with a variety of drugs. Good metabolic control probably reduces your risk of developing a neuropathy.

The reasons for the development of diabetic neuropathies is still not completely understood, but the overall cause is clearly higher-than-normal blood sugar. The ability of nerves to carry messages and the nature of the messages themselves may be altered by several chemical effects of poor control. The insulation of the nerves (the myelin sheath) is damaged. Sorbitol (a glucose-related alcohol) and fructose accumulate in nerve cells. The speed at which messages travel is slowed. Myo-inositol content of nerve tissues is reduced. (This deficiency may be corrected by drugs.) Glucose attaches to protein cells. The net result: a nerve disorder.

Neuropathies are caused by elevated blood sugar, so it is possible that good metabolic control will allow you to escape these complications and possibly reverse them if they develop. At this point, available evidence indicates that the possible benefits of optimal control are worth the cost.

The various forms of neuropathy are rare among young diabetics. They usually do not develop before fifteen years of diabetes. Generally, if the symptoms are mild in the first few years of neuropathy, they are unlikely to develop to an extreme degree.

Prevention

Maintain good metabolic control. Be aware that chemical toxins or alcoholic beverages may accelerate the development or progression of neuropathy.

Peripheral neuropathy

In this disorder, impairment occurs in those nerves extending down the legs and arms—the peripheral nervous system. Two main forms of disorders occur: those that develop gradually, usually without pain, and those with rapid onset and significant pain.

Gradual peripheral neuropathy is marked by numbness, tingling, itching, burning, a decreased sense of touch, a decrease in deep tendon reflexes, or any combination of these. These symptoms are usually found on both sides of the body and occur more frequently in the feet and legs than in the hands and arms. (Your doctor is checking for this disorder when testing your reflexes and when using the tuning fork and sharp devices to test your sensations.) Another possible symptom is the loss of the sense of orientation (proprioception) in the feet and legs—not knowing by feel which way a foot is turned, for instance.

While not painful, this form of nerve damage can lead to serious foot problems.

Treatment seems to be limited to improving control of diabetes. Myoinositol and sorbinil may prove to be effective against this form of neuropathy.

Peripheral neuropathy with rapid onset and pain is a temporary complication, but the pain can be intense. It develops within a matter of days or weeks and generally lasts from six to eighteen months. The chief symptom, a burning pain like a "toothache" in the feet or legs, is usually worse at night.

Treatment focuses on reducing the pain, first with aspirin or acetaminophen. Narcotics such as codeine, or drugs such as imipramine, Elavil or Prolixin may be used to provide relief. The anticonvulsant drugs, phenytoin or carbamazepine, although not substantiated in controlled clinical trials, may be worth a therapeutic trial. Some larger medical centers now have pain clinics offering a wide choice of treatments beyond drugs. Recently, capsaicin cream has helped nerve pain from skin contact that typically doesn't cause pain (like light touch, bedding, or clothes).

Autonomic neuropathy

This disorder affects the nerves controlling internal organs, genitals, small blood vessels and sweat glands of the skin, bladder muscles, and gastrointestinal tract. Some of the conditions that can result include impotence, difficulty urinating or sensing when the bladder is full (which can lead to bladder infection), diarrhea, stomach upset due to retention of food, dizziness after standing up, loss of the normal sweating response, and weakening or disappearance of the symptoms of an insulin reaction.

The symptoms of autonomic neuropathy are usually not temporary, as with some other forms of neuropathy. However, effective modes of treatment are available for most of the specific disabilities. Impotence from neuropathy, for instance, can be effectively overcome by a surgical implant that allows full sexual functioning. Several nonsurgical approaches, including external vacuum aids and drug injections, are also available. Tests are often given to distinguish clearly between neuropathic impotence and impotence caused by psychological factors, tests essential to avoiding unnecessary treatments.

We do not know to what extent metabolic control can reverse any of these conditions caused by autonomic neuropathy. Evidence so far indicates that stricter control can reverse the other form of neuropathy: peripheral.

Complications of the Feet and Legs

What goes wrong?

Two diabetic complications join forces to threaten the feet and legs of a diabetic: peripheral neuropathy and peripheral vascular disease. With proper self-care and regular foot examinations, you can neutralize this threat and reduce or eliminate the risk of losing a limb.

When peripheral neuropathy (described above) causes numbness and lack of feeling, injuries to the feet may go unnoticed, leading to infection and amputation. Pressure sores and ulcerations can develop on the feet and not be discovered until severe infection has set in.

328

This risk is compounded by the presence of peripheral vascular disease, a common disorder that takes a unique form with diabetes (described in this chapter under "Complications of the Heart and Circulatory System"). This disorder causes decreased blood flow in the legs and feet. This, in turn, means a decreased flow of the oxygen, white blood cells, and nutrients needed to fight infection. Either of the peripheral disorders can lead to loss. Together, the two multiply the risk.

One other foot problem can develop from lack of sensation. If any bone or joint disorders begin, symptoms may not be evident until they reach an advanced stage (neuroarthropathy). You are able to go on walking and standing without pain on feet and ankles that need immediate attention. This is not a common condition, but it is one more argument for excellent daily foot care.

Prevention of complications of the feet and legs

1. Maintain the best possible blood sugar control.

2. Do everything possible to prevent peripheral neuropathy, peripheral vascular disease, and hypertension.

3. Wash and inspect your feet daily. (If you can't see clearly or get close enough, have someone else do it for you.)

4. Check for blisters, bruises, cracks, cuts, and scratches. A sore, scratch, or red area that could be ignored by someone without diabetes should be watched very carefully by someone with diabetes. Use mild antiseptic and antibacterial salve on minor injuries. See your doctor for any sore that does not improve or heal within a few days. If the sore becomes infected or swollen, or if white or yellow pus appears, take no chances. See your doctor. You need to avoid serious infection, which can lead to gangrene and loss of a toe or foot.

5. Athlete's foot and fungal infections of the toenails should also be caught early and treated aggressively. Long-term care using antifungal creams or ointment may be necessary.

6. Massage your feet with anhydrous lanolin (available from your pharmacy) or polysorb. Do not rub lotion between the toes. (Massage helps maintain good circulation. Foot cream prevents dry, cracked skin.)

7. Do not cut or use patent medicines on corns or calluses. File calluses gently with an emery board. See your physician or a podiatrist for any large or painful lumps on your feet or for any changes in the shape of toes, toenails, or other parts of the foot.

8. When trimming toenails, gently round them to follow the shape of the toe. Avoid creating sharp points that dig into the next toe or sharp angles that cause ingrown toenails. Over-the-counter patent medicines for ingrown nails should also be avoided, as they may cause unwanted effects.

9. Select shoes that fit well and feel good. Break them in gradually. Always wear soft, seamless socks with shoes. Avoid sandals with thongs between the toes.

10. Inspect shoes daily for rocks, nail points, or damage.

11. Avoid very hot or very cold water. Do not use heating pads or hot water bottles on your feet. Wear socks to bed if your feet are cold.

12. Do foot and ankle exercises to stimulate circulation. (Two good exercises: rotating your feet at the ankle with your leg raised when you first wake up; standing with the front one-third of your feet on the edge of a step and raising and lowering your body a dozen times.)

13. Do not smoke. Nicotine is very damaging to the circulatory system.

Treatment

Early treatment of any foot disorder is essential, because infections can advance rapidly when circulation is poor. The primary guideline is to be alert and call or see your doctor for what may appear to be minor blisters, cuts or sores. The earlier these can be treated, the less likely they are to become serious.

Other Skin and Joint Complications

We want to mention briefly the thickening of the skin and possibly the connective tissue that may be present in up to one-third or more patients with insulin-dependent diabetes. It is usually painless and causes little if any disability. However, it can restrict joint movement, particularly in the wrists, hands, and fingers, and may be the cause of otherwise unexplained musculoskeletal problems. It can also affect the shoulder and neck. Because it is believed to result from glucose attaching itself to tissue proteins (AGEs), it may represent an early warning of other complications such as retinopathy, neuropathy, and nephropathy. The aldose reductase inhibitors may prove useful in relieving some of this limited joint mobility (LJM).

Less well known among medical professionals is the increased prevalence of frozen shoulder (adhesive capsulitis) among those with diabetes. In one large study, 11 percent of 800 patients with diabetes had frozen shoulder compared with 2.3 percent of 600 nondiabetic controls. If you notice any pain or limitation in the range of motion of your arm or shoulder, see your doctor. It is much easier to treat in the early stages (with stretching exercises or other physical therapy) than after it progresses.

Complications of the Heart and Circulatory System

In most cases, the characteristics of the following disorders are not unique to diabetes. We differ from nondiabetics only in having a higher risk for these problems, a risk that begins earlier in life (about ten years earlier). This risk can be reduced significantly by excellent self-care.

The primary risk factors for cardiovascular diseases (heart attack, stroke, arteriosclerosis, and peripheral vascular disease) are

- Smoking
- High fat and cholesterol levels in the blood
- Obesity
- Lack of exercise
- Family history of heart and circulatory disease
- High blood pressure

Prevention of cardiovascular disorders

A general preventive program for your heart and circulatory system includes may of the basic elements of the full diabetic regimen. Most of these are fundamental to a healthy life-style for anyone. They include the following:

1. Maintain normal body weight. If you are overweight, lose weight.

2. Limit sodium consumption to 2-4 grams per day if you have high blood pressure.

3. Avoid foods high in saturated fat and cholesterol.

4. Learn and use effective techniques of relaxation and stress reduction.

5. Exercise regularly, at an aerobic level if your condition allows.

6. If you smoke, stop smoking.

Since information on stroke and heart attacks is widely available, we will discuss only high blood pressure and peripheral vascular disease. These conditions have unique significance in diabetes.

High Blood Pressure

Prevention of chronically high blood pressure ranks close to blood sugar control as a means of avoiding diabetic complications. It also plays a major role in treatment of complications; lower blood pressure helps to slow or reverse the progress of eye, kidney, and circulatory problems. So here is a keystone of living well with diabetes: Act to maintain normal blood pressure before it starts to climb, and begin treatment promptly if it does go up.

What goes wrong?

Hypertension is more common among diabetics, and it tends to begin at an earlier age. The condition has no symptoms that you experience and can be diagnosed only through a series of blood pressure readings (consistent readings above 140/90). The causes of high blood pressure are not completely known. Contributing factors include obesity, stress, smoking, lack of activity, and genetic tendency.

Hypertension occurs more often in diabetics because high blood sugar and fats contribute to its development. Once narrowing of arteries due to fat deposits (atherosclerosis) or kidney disease start, these disorders further heighten blood pressure.

Although you feel no immediate symptoms, hypertension has very serious consequences for diabetics and nondiabetics alike. In any person, hypertension:

- Intensifies the buildup of fatty deposits, narrowing the blood vessels in a condition known as atherosclerosis, which increases all of the risks below.

- Causes your heart to work harder, enlarging it, and adding to your risk for heart attack.

- Increases your chances of developing peripheral vascular disease.

- Makes strokes more likely.

Diabetics have a higher risk for all of these disorders, a risk made even higher by hypertension. But there are further effects specific to diabetes. High blood pressure in diabetics also contributes to the development and progress of kidney disease and hastens the development of retinopathy.

Hypertension is called the silent disease, because its effects are not experienced directly. But it speaks loudly in its impact on our health.

Prevention

General preventive measures for circulatory disease are given at the beginning of this section. Following this set of recommendations is one of the greatest gifts you can give yourself, hundreds of times more valuable than the relatively small sacrifices involved.

Treatment

For a diabetic, when blood pressure consistently goes above 140/90, it is time to start treatment for hypertension. Fortunately, the first stage of treatment is to do the very things recommended for prevention, if you are not already doing them. You may not need medication,

333

assuming that your blood pressure is only mildly elevated and that other complications do not require it. You might want to buy a blood pressure cuff (sphygmomanometer), the device for measuring your blood pressure, so you can monitor your pressure at home between medical appointments.

If an antihypertensive drug is prescribed at the first sign of high blood pressure (and if you are willing to follow the recommendations above), ask your physician if there is any special reason to go directly to medication. If there is not, you both can consider a six-month trial to determine whether relaxation, sodium restriction, weight reduction, and so forth will bring your blood pressure down. Most people with high blood pressure need antihypertensive drugs, but if you can control blood pressure without them, you avoid the potential side effects of the drugs.

Great care must be taken in choosing an antihypertensive medication, as many of the products available have side effects potentially harmful to diabetics. Don't be afraid to ask your physician to choose the drug with the fewest possible side effects for you and your diabetes.

There are more than twenty-five different drugs available to lower blood pressure, including many new ones particularly useful for diabetics, such as ACE inhibitors. Some, however (propranolol and other beta blockers) eliminate the warning signs of an insulin reaction and block the release of the hormone that helps us recover from hypoglycemia. One of the most popular diuretics used for hypertension, hydrochlorothiazide, tends to increase both blood sugar and blood fat levels. Others reinforce the difficulties with impotence some diabetic men have. Adrenergic inhibitors are the worst offenders. These include reserpine, clonidine, and methyldopa.

You may feel uncomfortable raising the choice of drugs with your physician. We suggest that you say something like: "I've read that some of the common blood pressure drugs are not as good for diabetics as others. Can we discuss this? Which one(s) are you going to prescribe for me?" Most likely, the physician will respond with an explanation indicating an awareness of a considered choice and that more monitoring of blood sugar or potassium may be needed. Possible major side effects to watch for should be discussed,

If kidney disease has started, treatment for hypertension becomes more complex and even more important. High blood pressure hastens deterioration of kidney function. Kidney impairment further increases blood pressure. This vicious cycle can be slowed and possibly halted if medication and nondrug therapy are started early enough. Antihypertensive treatment and perhaps restriction of animal protein in your diet are the only factors believed to slow the advance of existing kidney disease. Under your physician's care, you should begin all of the measures listed in the general prevention of circulatory disease above. But you will need stricter control of salt in your diet (no more than 1 gram per day). The selection of drugs at this point is crucial and should be made by a physician familiar with diabetic kidney disorders.

Peripheral Vascular Disease

What goes wrong?

Poor circulation develops in the legs and feet of diabetics, mostly through atherosclerosis. The decreased blood flow results in inadequate supplies of oxygen and nutrients reaching cells in the feet. This is one of the major causes of the difficulties described under "Complications of the Feet and Legs." Disorders of this type can result in serious infection, gangrene and amputation. For this reason, foot care is one of the most vital aspects of your regimen.

Symptoms

Aching, cramping or pain sometimes occurs in the legs while walking. This pain usually subsides in a few minutes when you rest. (Its technical name is intermittent claudication.) Other symptoms are

- Cold feet.
- Aching in the legs or feet when lying down.
- Feet that become red or purplish when your legs hang down.
- Pulses in the feet that become weaker, particularly after a brisk walk.
- Feet that become pale when raised above your body.
- Reduced blood pressure at the ankles.

Prevention

The basic cardiovascular preventive measures described all apply here. You should also review and follow the foot care recommendations given under "Complications of the Feet and Legs."

Treatment

Treatment of peripheral vascular disease seeks to avoid the consequences of poor circulation. Pentoxifylline may help to relieve symptoms. Surgery to bypass the diseased blood vessels or angioplasty to open them up may be necessary for severe persistent pain.

Summary

Complications are the most disturbing aspect of having diabetes. We face serious risks, and it is still unclear how much we can actually do to prevent complications from developing. Yet we can defy this uncertainty and face the consequences of diabetes bravely, even if we do develop a complication. We are free to reduce the risks and improve our odds.

We are, after all, individuals, each with our own unique history. Some of us will live long lives without major complications. Others will delay the onset and lessen the severity of the disorders that result from diabetes. Ever-improving treatment of these afflictions will enable us to limit their consequences in our lives. By learning to follow the balanced and healthy life-style this book presents, we will be able to live well with diabetes, even if its complications develop.

BOOKS ON DISEASES OF THE HEART AND BLOOD VESSELS

Dr. Dean Ornish's Program for Reversing Heart Disease, Random House, New York (1990).

Heartcare, rev. ed. American Medical Association. Random House, New York (1984).

Your Heart: Questions You Have...Answers You Need. Ed Weiner. Peoples Medical Society, Emmaus, Penn. (1985).

Take Care of Your Heart: The Complete Book of Heart Facts. E. A. Amsterdam and A. M. Holmes. Facts on File Publications, New York (1984).

Heart to Heart: Cleveland Clinic Guide to Understanding Heart Disease and Open Heart Surgery. N. V. Richards. Atheneum, New York (1987).

Coming Back—A Guide to Recovering from a Heart Attack rev. ed. K. Cohn and D. Duke. Addison Wesley, Reading, Mass. (1987).

There is no single book that covers the entire field of heart disease adequately. Look for these or other books in your local library or bookstore.

Section VI
WOMEN AND CHILDREN LIVING WELL

Living Well As A Diabetic Woman

This chapter was written by Cathy Feste for the first edition. We have edited it minimally and brought it up to date. Cathy is a nationally recognized health motivation specialist, president of her own wellness consulting business, and the author of the best-selling book The Physician Within. She has had insulin-dependent diabetes for more than thirty years.

As a woman who has lived with diabetes for thirty-five years, I know that it carries with it some special challenges. I have seen my blood sugars swoop when a period is approaching. I saw my insulin requirements nearly quadruple during my pregnancy. As I nursed my baby, I faced the additional challenges of low blood sugar as my body burned extra calories.

Those are physical issues. But there's another side to life with diabetes. Being unwilling to miss out on the fun and fulfillment of life has required extra creativity. As a teenager, I found that cheerleading and marching band worked out fine if I hid LifeSavers in my uniform.

Girl Scout canoe trips were not a problem if I kept insulin, syringes, testing strips, and carbohydrates in airtight plastic containers that would float. These early successes gave me the confidence as an adult to ski in the Rocky Mountains.

Living well as a diabetic woman requires adapting to certain physical requirements without sacrificing the quality of life. It's a constant balancing act. This chapter discusses the major physical issues unique to women with diabetes. It also explores some emotional and spiritual concerns associated with the disease.

PHYSICAL ISSUES

Diabetes presents women with special challenges during pregnancy, menstruation, and menopause. The interactions between blood sugar and hormone levels during these times affect our blood glucose regulation. Control, in turn, has a profound effect on pregnancy. Awareness of these effects will help you to manage both your diabetes and these aspects of your womanhood.

Menstruation

Interviews with both diabetic women and doctors reveal that, although hormones affect blood glucose levels, the effect is not uniform in all women. Even more frustrating is the fact that the effect can vary in the same woman; some months the blood sugars may rise dramatically, and some months they fall. Living well with the hormonal challenge requires a team effort. It is important for you to have medical advisors on your team who are knowledgeable and experienced in diabetes as well as female issues. They will best understand the general effect of hormones on blood sugars. Your job as a member of the team will be to record blood glucose levels accurately before, during, and after your menstrual periods. If you find a definite pattern, then together you can determine an appropriate course of action. If, for example, your blood sugar levels are consistently high the week before your period begins, then you may be able to successfully anticipate the increased need for insulin. However, it may not be that easy if you needs cannot be anticipated. The hormonal impact may vary or your periods may be inconsistent.

There is an individualized and changeable hormonal impact on blood sugar levels. Your choices are as follows. (1) With the help of your medical advisors, make a monthly plan of action designed to anticipate and meet your needs. (2) Do nothing anticipatory, but deal with the fluctuating blood sugars with the same strategies you use to cope with any stress-related, unpredictable blood sugars.

In addition, remember the strategy used by every woman in dealing with a period: When you can't exactly predict when it's coming, you start carrying some form of protection with you toward the end of the month so that you're prepared when it starts. We get frustrated and angry about periods when we are not prepared for them. The same is true of diabetes. Insulin reactions or high sugar levels are far more frustrating to us when we are ill prepared to handle them. When we handle them well, we increase our entire sense of well-being.

Birth Control

Since blood glucose should be under control before a woman becomes pregnant, it is important that a woman with diabetes practice birth control as soon as she becomes sexually active. Various methods are available. The method of choice will be determined through careful consideration of its effect on the woman's health as well as her personal preference.

In her book *The Diabetic Woman,* Dr. Lois Jovanovic-Peterson recommends that if a woman does not have high blood pressure, she may use low-dose birth control pills. Their impact on insulin doses is minimal. Dr. Jovanovic-Peterson writes that research shows that birth control pills do not increase the risk of blood clots. (Women with diabetic retinopathy should seek the advice of a specialist in diabetic retinopathy.) Dr. Jovanovic-Peterson points out, however, that some women will require higher-dose pills that do affect glucose and insulin requirements.

If birth control pills are not chosen, women can use barrier methods such as the diaphragm, condom, or cervical sponge. Talk this over with a trusted medical advisor.

Pregnancy

"When I decided to get married, my physician said to me: 'I think it's fine if you get married. But don't ever have children. Don't spread your genes around.' Because I am an educator, I believe that people ought to be given information and then make their own decisions. I felt that this doctor was giving me his personal opinion rather than information upon which to make a very important decision. So, my husband and I saw a genetic counselor who gave us not only information, but also a great deal of encouragement about the genetic issues involved. Appropriately informed about genetic issues and my good health, my husband and I choose to have a baby."

The outcome of diabetic pregnancies has improved dramatically. Many years ago, women with diabetes had miscarriages at an alarmingly higher rate than did their nondiabetic counterparts. Today, a healthy woman with diabetes can expect an outcome similar to that of the general population if

1. She is seen and closely followed by a knowledgeable medical team experienced in diabetic pregnancies. Teams vary from center to center, but they usually include specialists in endocrinology, diabetology, obstetrics, dietetics, nursing, psychology, and social work or family counseling.

2. She is educated about caring for diabetes and is motivated to act on what she learns.

3. Her diabetes is under control *before* she becomes pregnant.

4. She keeps blood glucose levels within normal limits throughout the pregnancy. Research indicates that babies in utero tolerate low blood sugars much better than they tolerate high blood sugars.

The mother's health should be assessed before she conceives. If she has existing complications, especially of the kidney and eye, she must be informed about what effects the pregnancy might have on her health and the health of her baby. After an evaluation by a doctor extensively educated and experienced in both diabetes and pregnancy, the potential mother can make an informed choice about whether or not to attempt a pregnancy.

Ask your physician how many diabetic pregnancies he or she has managed. Also ask for a description of how your physician manages diabetic pregnancies. You need to have an obstetrician and a diabetes care specialist who are knowledgeable and experienced with diabetic pregnancies. If you know of no such physicians, ask your local American Diabetes Association chapter for a referral.

Another essential element of a successful pregnancy is good health insurance. Even an uncomplicated diabetic pregnancy includes extra tests and visits to the medical team. A complicated pregnancy could include a lengthy hospitalization as well as intensive neonatal care for the baby. Make sure you have good health insurance before you become pregnant.

Throughout pregnancy, you should keep your blood sugars as nearly normal as possible. Chapter 5 of this book provides detailed information for learning the intensive regimen needed for this level of control. Your doctor will adapt this regimen to your individual needs. Besides the impact on the overall successful outcome of a pregnancy, it is important to keep blood sugars in normal range for the sake of the baby's size. The pregnant mother's blood sugar crosses the placenta. When the sugars are high, the baby's pancreas produces insulin to normalize them. In the process of using the mother's blood sugar, the baby gains weight. The baby's weight is one of the factors that determines the method through which the baby is delivered. Babies of normal weight can be delivered vaginally if the health of both the mother and the baby is otherwise good. Large babies must be delivered by Caesarean section.

Close blood sugar control presents numerous challenges. Ironically, close control increases the risk of severe insulin reactions (hypoglycemia). Fortunately, this is not a great problem for the baby, since babies can tolerate low blood sugar much better than high. The risk of low blood sugar is to the mother and her diabetes management. One undesirable result of low blood sugar is a swing to high blood sugar (hyperglycemia) and a bouncing effect that can upset one's control for a day or longer. Testing blood sugars more frequently is an excellent strategy for avoiding hypoglycemia.

One reason blood sugars rise too high following a low-blood-sugar episode is that people sometimes eat more than they need to counteract the lower sugar level.

> *"While I was pregnant, I forced myself to drink four ounces of juice and then wait a full fifteen minutes before taking anything more if the symptoms had not subsided. To help me wait, I pretended that it was a middle-of-the-night feeding for the baby. I viewed this strategy of treating low blood sugar as good practice for motherhood."*

With self blood glucose monitoring, we now have tools to tell us the impact of the food we eat. This is especially helpful when we need to assess the impact on low blood sugar. After you have eaten, you should wait fifteen minutes before rechecking blood sugar. After fifteen minutes, if the reading is still low and has not moved toward normal levels, drink another glass of juice or milk and retest in another fifteen minutes.

Doing periodic 3:00 a.m. blood tests can help to prevent problems with very low blood sugars. Report middle-of-the-night low blood sugars to your doctor. A change in your insulin dosage may be required. You may already be doing 3:00 a.m. blood tests on days when you are unusually active and are more inclined to an ongoing blood sugar-lowering effect. Knowing your body and your unique responses to activity, food, and stress is extremely helpful.

Close control of blood sugars will mean that your life-style during pregnancy will be closely regulated. This may not be typical of your usual way of living. Most of us slide off our regimens occasionally, and some do so fairly frequently. Reflect carefully on your willingness to maintain tight control in order to have a responsible pregnancy. Although it does require effort on the part of the diabetic woman, many women have reported that it actually turned out to be less of a challenge than they had anticipated. A common comment from pregnant women with diabetes is that their growing abdomen serves as a constant reminder of why they're working so hard.

> *"I made a commitment to follow my diabetic regimen to a point of perfection. Neither birthday nor any other holiday suc-*

ceeded in tempting me to deviate from my meal plan. I related to a cartoon I saw just before Christmas. Two little boys in a department store were standing before a Christmas display. One boy said to the other, 'I'm so good at this time of year I can hardly stand myself.' While I understood that feeling, I also made the surprising discovery that it actually became easier and easier simply to make no exceptions. And I had a tremendous amount of support from the medical team.

The team of mother, father, obstetrician, diabetologist, dietitian, and nurse worked hard to make my pregnancy successful. I was extremely thankful to have an upbeat, 'human' medical team whose humor and warmth reinforced the excitement of a pregnancy instead of treating it like a high-risk, complicated medical problem. Whenever the seriousness of the situation did arise, I felt supported rather than fearful. For example, my diabetes doctor told me that any sign of infection, high sugars, or ketones should be reported immediately and not be left until tomorrow. It wasn't frightening to hear him say that, just reassuring to know that he would be there to help.

Besides wonderful medical support, I was blessed with a supportive husband who gave me a steady diet of love and humor. As my abdomen increased, I began to wonder how much longer I should inject my insulin abdominally. Although my obstetrician gave me the answer 'as long as it is both physically and psychologically comfortable,' it was my husband's response that took the prize. He told me, 'Just keep injecting in your abdomen until you hear someone say 'ouch.' ' Humor gives wonderful perspective."

Laboratory tests are an important part of support in a diabetic pregnancy. Each test and each visit to your medical team is an excellent reminder that you are not alone. Skilled people are doing everything they can to help you.

The baby's birth does not signify the end of the close working relationship between the mother and medical team. If you choose to nurse your baby, you must be well informed about your caloric needs for milk production as well as the ongoing balancing act with insulin.

Throughout pregnancy, insulin requirements increase. Toward the end of a pregnancy, a woman may be taking two to three times as much insulin as in her prepregnancy days. At the time of birth, insulin requirements drop dramatically and a woman becomes extremely sensitive to insulin. Some women require no insulin immediately following delivery. The nursing mother may drop bedtime insulin entirely as her body burns many calories overnight for the production of milk. The teamwork continues. The baby is its newest member.

Because information on diabetic pregnancies is continually changing and growing, we encourage you to rely more on your medical advisors than on any printed information. Reflect on the issues. Make informed, responsible choices.

To Pregnant Women Whose Diabetes Is Not in Good Control...

The advice given so far on preparing for a diabetic pregnancy may raise fears in anyone who is already pregnant and maintaining less-than-excellent blood glucose control. Have you endangered either your baby's health or your own? There is no simple answer. You must discuss your situation with an obstetrician experienced in diabetic pregnancies.

In the past, when tight control was not yet possible, many women had successful pregnancies with only minor difficulties. Statistically, these women and their babies were in greater risk, but each individual pregnancy had its own outcome. Even if your control has been moderate to poor, you may still have few problems if you regulate your blood glucose levels now. Discuss this fully with your medical team.

Beyond this, you may want to explore the techniques for working through possible resistance to maintaining good control in Chapters 3 and 14.

Vaginitis

Some women report that their diabetes was diagnosed when they went to see their doctor about severe vaginal itching. This problem is usually due to yeast infection. Diabetic women have an increased incidence of yeast infections because yeast grows more rapidly in glucose. The infections occur more frequently when blood sugars are high enough that glucose is present in the urine. Your doctor can prescribe treatments for yeast infections, but prevention is better. Generally these infections can be prevented by keeping the urine free of sugar.

Recently, a well-controlled study showed that eating 8 ounces of yogurt daily decreased the number of yeast present in the vagina as well as the number of yeast infections. It is important to make sure that the yogurt you buy in the market contains live (not pasteurized) *lactobacilli acidophilus*. The L. acidophilus presumably directly inhibits yeast growth and survival. (Clearly, this treatment is great if you like yogurt. Of course, you must count the yogurt in your diet.)

If you choose to keep blood sugars in a normal range, refer to Chapter 5, "The Intensive Regimen." Using this chapter as a guide, discuss improving your regimen with your physician.

Menopause

At some point in middle age, women cease having periods. Because certain hormones are no longer present, the need for insulin usually drops. However, if the hormones are replaced, then insulin requirements will be affected by the estrogen and progesterone. According to Dr. Lois Jovanovic-Peterson, a noted authority in diabetic women's issues and herself a diabetic, the insulin requirements with hormone replacement are determined by how closely the hormone doses match the woman's needs. Higher doses of hormones requires higher doses of insulin.

Day-to-day variations during menopause are far easier to handle with blood glucose monitoring. Some women experience profuse sweating during menopause and wonder if it is caused by hypoglycemia or by their "change." With blood testing, a woman can generally figure out what's happening and get in control of her life.

Hormones do affect blood sugar levels. You can choose whether or not to take hormones. Since a history of cancer is another factor to consider in making this decision, it is best to discuss all the factors with your carefully selected medical advisors. Remember that you are a unique person, and the effect your hormones have on your blood sugar levels may be different from what you hear from other women or read about. When books describe what is *normal*, they are more accurately describing what is *average*. Since few of us are "average," you should work with your medical team to understand your unique reactions. Doing this is another leg of the journey toward personal growth and fulfillment.

It is comforting to have support for the physical needs of diabetes— the timing of meals, appropriate food, and time and space for monitoring blood glucose. But there is another type of support that is equally important, if not more so. That is emotional support.

EMOTIONAL ISSUES

I believe that women who have diabetes have a distinct advantage over men who have diabetes. Traditionally, women have found it easier to connect with friends on an emotional level. To receive emotional support, one needs to understand the language and be willing to engage in the process of both seeking and receiving it. The language of emotional support includes "I feel...I need...I am angry, fearful, lonely because..." "It makes me feel so good when..." Getting emotional support includes a willingness to begin conversations with phrases like these. The process also requires time and an appropriate setting. A fifteen-minute commute on the way to work won't do it. A meeting in a relaxed atmosphere like a restaurant or your home, with an hour's worth of time, is more likely to allow the process to work.

People who feel reticent to begin talking with their friends about the feelings they have about diabetes may find it very helpful to attend a meeting of the local American Diabetes Association. Meeting others who have diabetes often creates an instantaneous bond that connects people on an emotional level.

A variety of support groups are available to people who are interested in group interaction. At many ADA chapters, visitation programs are now being offered. These allow people who have diabetes and are feeling "stuck" to meet one-to-one with others who have diabetes. This effective program provides two-way benefit, as both the giver and the recipient find support. If this type of program appeals to you, check with your local ADA chapter or affiliate. Whether it's through a formalized program of social support or the casual warmth of two friends having coffee, take the step toward connecting on a feeling level. It may seem awkward at first, but keep at it. The rewards are great.

Dating and Marriage

Some women are reluctant to tell their dates that they have diabetes. If you are dating, consider the following scenarios.

1. Which situation would be better?

    a. You have an insulin reaction when you are with a man who knows you have diabetes.

    b. You have a reaction when you are with someone who hasn't a clue as to why your behavior is changed.

2. You are dating someone who needs to eat at a particular time. Would you prefer to have your date tell you that? Or, would you prefer to have him jeopardize his health to eat a fashionably late dinner?

3. Do you really believe that diabetes is such an awful disease that someone would not want to date you because of it?

    a. If your answer is yes, you should talk to a diabetes educator who can help you to adapt to diabetes and have a fun and full social life.

    b. If your answer is no, remember that you can influence the way your date thinks about diabetes. Present it positively, as a disease that can be controlled through a healthy life-style.

    "A touching and reinforcing moment for me came at a party, one evening when I overhead my husband say to the group of people with whom he was visiting: 'The best thing that ever happened to me was marrying someone with diabetes. We live such a healthy life.'

Dating was not particularly problematic for me in terms of my diabetes until marriage became an issue. It is at major decision points in life—such as marriage, career, children—that one is confronted again with accepting the fact that diabetes, like any chronic disease, is unavoidably a part of life and of that decision.

While my husband and I were dating, I wondered about what diabetes would mean for him if we were married. But I did like his attitude. He was at ease—never treating me like a 'diabetic,' but rather as an attractive (to him) young woman. And he had just the right measure of concern; that is, he asked questions about appropriate restaurant choice, timing of meals, and what, if any, dessert I would eat when we ate at his parents' house for the first time. Humor helped us through the rough spots (and it still does!).

But somewhere in my subconscious a shadow was lurking, and I couldn't quite make out what it meant. A wonderfully sensitive physician helped me bring it into the light so that I could see it and deal with it. It was this: Just before I became engaged, I visited my doctor. In the waiting room, I met a young woman exactly my age who was losing her sight as a result of diabetes.

Suddenly I had an urgent need to know the future. I wanted my doctor to look into a crystal ball and tell me what course my diabetes would take, so that I would have some idea of what 'for better or worse' might mean to my husband. My doctor gently explained to me that no one knows what the future will bring. Perhaps the most profound lesson that diabetes has taught me is this: Diabetes does not make life any more uncertain. It simply makes us more aware of the uncertainty of life."

People blessed with the awareness that life is uncertain are in a unique position to enjoy life more fully. Time is more likely to be savored than wasted. All of life's experiences become a potential source of wonder. The embarrassment of saying "I love you" gives way to appreciation for having the courage to say it.

It is helpful to be able to identify what makes your life fulfilling, because that's what will motivate you to handle any challenge that threatens your enjoyment of life. Your desire to live fully will mobilize the great inner strengths that you have.

"My husband and I wed and have enjoyed healthy, happy times. Four years after we married, we had a child. I knew that our son would never see his mother coping with stress by taking alcohol or drugs. My early experiences had already set healthy stress-management habits of diet and activity.

Our family life has been full. I have felt great and participated actively and fully in my teaching career as well as having a social life of partying, cross-country skiing, and bicycling."

Most women fully expect to enjoy retirement with their husbands. They also expect to watch every hockey game of their children as they grow up. They look forward to graduations, weddings, and grandchildren. Without the challenge of a chronic disease, it is easier to deny that untimely death could ever rob them of their lifelong plans. Besides a mighty important lesson about the uncertainty of life, diabetes can give one the gift of appreciating how precious life is. It's an odd and profound gift that is difficult to explain. It's like appreciating the fragile, exquisite beauty of a snowflake with the understanding that it may be the last one you'll ever see along with the faith that it isn't. Perhaps the oddest part of the gift is the realization that we receive this gift through suffering. The painful awareness of our mortality actually gives us the gift of appreciating life.

Balancing the Emotions

Although there surely are times when diabetes causes us to grapple with life's most profound issues, there are plenty of times when having diabetes is little more than a minor inconvenience. Balancing the emotions of those very different viewpoints is important to one's overall well-being.

"At about the six-week point in my pregnancy (before it had been confirmed), I attend a diabetes and pregnancy conference. It was directed to health professionals and contained (to me, because I suspected I was pregnant) a ton of horror. I heard someone talk about the possibility of brain damage to the baby if ketones were

present in the early weeks of development. That horrified me because I had been experiencing fasting ketosis recently. I went to my doctor immediately following the conference. He explained that in the early weeks of fetal development the body's need for calories greatly increases, and that's why I had ketones in my urine. An increase in calories and insulin took care of the physical problems.

I resolved to avoid similar conferences during my pregnancy to alleviate my emotional discomfort. But this is not to recommend ignorance as bliss. Education is a most important ally. I sincerely believe that one must strive for the balance of knowing what you need to know and then avoiding a mental diet of facts that only frighten and immobilize the spirit. I knew that my carefully selected physicians knew the facts, dangers, and cautions of a diabetic pregnancy. I allowed them to do the worrying. I concentrated my efforts on doing all that they recommended and then did everything possible to keep mind and spirit positive and hopeful."

To follow a self-care regimen, we need to accept the seriousness of diabetes as well as our personal vulnerability. Then, we also need hope. We need to understand all of our options for health and act on them. Reflect on the issues that cause you emotional discomfort. Talk them over with a trusted advisor. Act to prevent problems, and promote health and well-being. By taking positive action, you will gain an overall sense of control over your life.

CAREER CONCERNS

Until the mid-eighties, women were bombarded with advice about what to do with their lives. We were urged to seek nontraditional careers. We were told to rebel against being "just homemakers." But now the pendulum seems to be swinging toward more reasonable advice: Women should be able to choose whatever they want to do— have a career, go to school, stay at home, do volunteer work, or combine any of these choices. If the choices they make are manageable and fulfilling, women can find satisfaction and harmony in their lives. If they undertake either too little or too much, the effects are negative and stressful. Balance is essential to anyone who wants a happy, healthy life. We need enough meaningful activity to give life excitement and a sense of purpose, but not so much activity that we are overwhelmed by demands on us. All men and women struggle with this balancing of life. When diabetes is present, it is simply another ball to juggle.

Reflect on your own life challenges as I share a few of mine.

Diabetes goes with me:

- Into the hospital where I do volunteer work. I attend monthly meetings from 4:00 until 6:00 p.m. To keep balance, I do a blood test just before the meeting and then help myself to the fruit and crackers offered if I need them. My own supply of dried fruit is ever at hand should I need more.

- On national and international airplane flights. I juggle time-zone changes and insulin requirements according to my doctor's good advice. With snacks like dried fruit and granola bars in my purse or briefcase, I can cope when a meal flight ends up serving no food. I always carry my blood glucose meter with me on the plane. Extra tests reassure me that I am remaining in balance.

- Up to the podium as I make presentations. A blood test before speaking tells me if my jitters are simply from nervousness or if I am hypoglycemic.

- Into those "one-hour" meetings that begin at 11:00 a.m. and end at 1:00 p.m. Inconspicuous snacks like LifeSavers keep me going without interrupting the meeting.

Diabetes is ever present when I'm working too many hours and forgetting to balance my work with exercise (for the body). I have seen tests of 400 as a result of the distress of imbalance. It is tempting to curse my diabetes, saying "If it weren't for that darned diabetes, I could keep up the same pace as my friends do!" But then I look at the picture more carefully. What is really happening is this: Diabetes tells me when life is out of balance and my body is asking me not to abuse it. Diabetes, in this case, is a blessing in disguise. In fact, I often find myself cautioning my nondiabetic friends to take better care of themselves. Although they know the harmful effects of stress, they don't have a tool (like my blood glucose meter) to tell them that their stress is harming them.

IN MY HEART OF HEARTS...

The heart of life is neither male or female, for it beats for all. The skills we need to live well with diabetes are the very same skills that anyone needs to meet the inevitable pain and challenges of life. To experience joy and soul-satisfying growth, we need to believe that diabetes has that gift to give. Great philosophers teach us that pain hollows us out, allowing us to hold more joy. They even suggest that pain holds as much wonder as joy. Indeed, joy and sorrow are inseparable in the same way that pain and growth often come together.

With maturity, we all become philosophers to some degree. If we can accept the philosophy that pain brings growth, then we have the foundation upon which to build a healthy life. Neitzche said that people who have a *why* to life can bear almost any *how*. With this belief, we accept diabetes as one more building block of life.

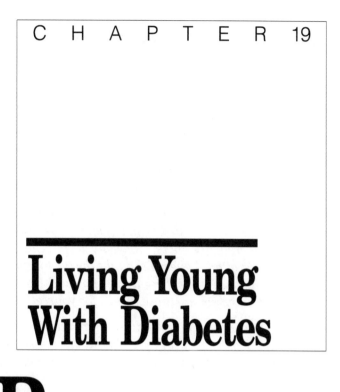

CHAPTER 19

Living Young With Diabetes

Believe it or not, every grown-up has a child inside that remembers what being a kid is all about. The authors of this book asked the kids inside them to write about having diabetes when they were young. Cathy was 10, Gary was 12, and Ernie was 14 when their diabetes started.

You're really lucky to be a kid now. The doctors and nurses today know so much more about diabetes than when we were kids. They're good at helping you learn all the things you need to know about taking care of yourself. They've finally figured out that kids can do all kinds of complex things, like testing their own blood sugar. Children are a lot smarter than most grown-ups probably realize.

Having diabetes keeps us on our toes—more than most people. Some great entertainers and athletes have diabetes. Wade Wilson, Mary Tyler Moore, and Catfish Hunter have diabetes, and it hasn't stopped them. It doesn't have to stop you. With diabetes or without diabetes, there is a world of things we can accomplish if we really want to.

The kid inside Ernie says:

> *One dumb thing I had to get over when I was a kid was pretending not to have diabetes. For a long time, I ate whatever I wanted (usually when no one was looking). I even forgot shots and ended up in the hospital in a coma one time. I thought if I acted like I didn't have diabetes, it would just go away. But it didn't.*
>
> *I think I would have been a lot happier if I had taken better care of myself. I don't mean being perfect! But I wish I had remembered my shots, done my tests regularly, and not eaten sweets so often. I guess I thought the doctor and my mom and dad were the ones I did these things for, and I resented them for that. Now I know you do those things for yourself, not for anybody else.*
>
> *Sometimes having diabetes makes me feel sad or angry or afraid. Don't ever think you shouldn't have these feelings. They are a natural part of you, and there's no reason to pretend you don't have them. When I kept my feelings inside, I ended up doing things that were worse than saying "I'm angry."*

The kid inside Gary says:

> *My doctor wanted me to meet another young person with diabetes while I was still in the hospital. (When I was a kid, you had to stay in the hospital for several days just to get regulated). I was embarrassed to meet this person. It was even worse because he was coming to the hospital just to see me. I don't remember his name, but he was just a little older than me and he seemed nice. I remember him telling me that taking insulin gets to be a habit, like brushing our teeth. It helped me to talk to someone else who had diabetes. It took away some of my fear. At the time, I didn't think it was that important. But I still remember it.*
>
> *In a way, diabetes really helped me grow up. I learned about taking responsibility. I learned how to talk about diabetes and even other things without being ashamed. I learned how to talk to the coaches at school and the dietitian in the school kitchen. I learned how to arrange my life so that diabetes didn't interfere too much. I learned how to go out with my friends and do what they did and still keep my diabetes under pretty good control.*

The kid inside Cathy says:

When I was little, they didn't even have blood sugar testing you could do at home. Blood tests are a lot better than testing your urine. They help you know if you have enough energy for playing hard without having reactions. But remember, those test numbers are just facts to help you. They don't say whether you're a good person or a bad person. They just tell what your blood sugar is, so you can figure out how to change your insulin, food, or exercise.

It's a little like being a scientist. If your blood sugar is higher or lower than you want it to be, you can usually figure out why. Maybe you ran extra hard today. Maybe your snack was bigger than usual. Maybe you've got a bad cold. When you figure out the reason your blood sugars are off, you're not only a scientist, you're a detective, too!

My doctor first told me I had diabetes when I was in the hospital for a broken arm. A clown came to my room to cheer me up and give me a balloon. I said, "I just have a broken arm and diabetes. I'm not sick!" I went on feeling that way and never saw diabetes as a reason not to do anything. I did everything my friends did, except for eating a lot of sweet things.

I asked my mom if having diabetes would make me different from the other kids. She told me, "You'll be stronger and more in charge of your life. You'll learn how to take care of yourself and eat the right things. That will mean our whole family will benefit because we'll learn to take care of ourselves from you.

All three of us say:

We know having diabetes is a problem sometimes, but we want you to remember that having diabetes doesn't mean you're sick. You just have to watch some things other kids don't ever have to think about. (Some people think that makes us smarter than other people.) But most of the things we are supposed to do are healthy for everybody.

You'll be learning about diabetes for a long time, probably the rest of your life. We hope there will be a cure for you to learn about someday. Scientists are working on it now, but nobody's sure when they'll find it. Until they do, take good care of yourself so the cure will work for you.

TO THE PARENTS OF A DIABETIC YOUTH...

Credo for the parent of a diabetic child

My child is an essentially healthy person who happens to have some qualities that need special attention, not a sick child who must be protected.

My child is capable of learning to handle all aspects of diabetes care over time, not someone who must remain dependent on me.

My child will learn to take good care of diabetes by following my model of healthful behavior and by receiving positive rewards, not from threats of the consequences of diabetes.

I will find the right balance between my responsibility as a parent and my child's growing responsibility for his or her own life, including the care of diabetes.

When I feel I can't cope, I will get the help I need to go on living well and aiding my child to live well. I do not need to sacrifice my life to diabetes.

To live well with childhood diabetes calls for a unique partnership between you and your child, one that can enrich and deepen your relationship. You can learn together, adapt together, and feel together as you meet the demands of this condition. With a preteen, especially, you become an authoritative source of information and guidance as you learn about diabetes. At the same time, you respect and support your child's growing capacity for self-management and participation in decision making.

Having a child with diabetes presents enough special challenges that you deserve a book specifically addressing your child's and your unique needs. Fortunately, there is an excellent one that we suggest you get if you are the parent of a diabetic youth. It was written by the founder of the Juvenile Diabetes Foundation, Lee Ducat, who is herself the parent of a diabetic. You can find a complete reference and description of this book at the end of this chapter, together with several other resources specific to parents and youth.

We begin with an often-neglected subject: your own needs as the parent of a youth with diabetes.

Take Care of Yourself!

Many of the techniques for living well described in this book apply to your life as well as your child's. Your maintenance of psychological health, good diet, and exercise programs become a model for your child. This is the very best way of teaching—to be what you want your child to become. With this understanding, taking care of yourself helps both you and your child. And you avoid the useless martyr role— sacrificing yourself for someone else's well-being.

Use the tips for stress management and coping included in Chapters 3, 11, and 14, and find a support group for parents of diabetics through your local chapter of the American Diabetes Association. Parents with experience can help you cope with your problems and guide you in handling the problems that come up with your child. (See Chapter 13 for more on support groups and networks for both you and your child.)

Adapting the Living Well Approach to Your Child's Situation

The underlying approach of this book is respect for the capacity of the individual person with diabetes to make wise self-care choices. We believe the diabetes regimen must be individualized; that adherence to it grows when parental attention is positive rather than threatening; and that living well is a matter of one's whole life, not just blood sugar levels.

As the parent of a child or teenager, you may wonder if these beliefs are fully applicable without risk to your child. Can a child of 5 or 6 make wise choices to handle precise techniques like insulin injections or home blood glucose testing? What will control the rebelliousness of your teen other than threats of future catastrophes if he or she doesn't shape up?

Many parents and diabetic youths have demonstrated this approach by sharing responsibility fully, discussing decisions together, and gradually passing responsibility on to the growing child. Children as young as 5 have learned to use meters accurately to test blood sugar levels and to give their own insulin. Rebelliousness may be an inevitable part of the teen years, but there is little evidence that coercion and threats are an effective way of handling it. The *Living Well* approach gives a teenager positive reinforcement and opportunities to learn to make more responsible choices.

Balance and Individualization

We have emphasized the need to design a diabetes treatment program specific to the needs and character of the individual throughout this book. Now we must consider two or three individuals—the child and the parents—as well as the rest of the family. Living well with youthful diabetes demands a balance between lives of all the family members and an adaptation to the unique pattern of the individual family.

Different families have very different patterns concerning responsibility, decision making, participation, emotional support, health practices, and other areas important to diabetes care. You must find a way of dealing with the demands of diabetes that fits your family's patterns. But you may need to change patterns that unintentionally undermine your child's ability to live well. He or she may find it difficult to follow a healthful life-style if the rest of the family eats an unhealthy diet, doesn't exercise, and handles stress poorly. Becoming responsible for his or her own care will be hard if the parents are either too protective or too dominating.

My Family Profile

To identify your family's patterns, explore your answers to this questionnaire. You can gain insight into your own family's patterns and how they may affect your diabetic youth.

1. How are decisions made in your family?_____

   _____

   Do you discuss issues together?_____

   _____

Do you explore alternative options to choose from?_____

Who participates in the actual decision making?_____

What matters do the children decide on their own?_____

In what areas are the children simply given orders?_____

2. How well do the children follow either their own decisions or suggestions, and orders given by parents?

Parent's opinions_____

Children's opinions_____

How well do the parents follow either their own decisions or directions given by external authority?_____

3. When a child disobeys or acts irresponsibly, how do the parents respond?_____

What is done to help the child act differently?_____

Do these things work?_____

4. In your family who has taken the responsibility to learn about diabetes?_____

Mother_____ Father _____ Child _____

5. Does the family as a whole follow a healthful life-style?_____

   A moderate and balanced diet?_____

   Regular exercise and activity?_____

   Effective stress management?_____

   Emotional stability?_____

6. What major challenges other than diabetes face you and your family?_____

Your answers may suggest areas where your family could strengthen its ability to cope with diabetes and other life challenges. Parents can use the results of this exercise to discuss possible changes, first between themselves and then with the whole family.

AGES AND PHASES OF YOUTHFUL DIABETES

The age of your child will determine how you adapt this book to your situation. In this section, we will make a few suggestions for different ages.

Infancy to Age 4 or 5

If you have a young child with diabetes, *Living Well* will be a major educational source for you, but you will need guidance in many aspects of caring for and educating your child. Your health care team and diabetes support network will play an important role, even more than with older children. The Introduction and Chapter 1 offer basic attitudes and practices that you can draw on in your parenting. Chapters 3, 11, and 14 will help you help yourself as well as your child with the emotional challenges of diabetes. Toward the end of this phase, you can cautiously begin sharing responsibility for day-to-day diabetes tasks. As the young one demonstrates expertise under your supervision, you will gain confidence and a sense of what he or she can handle.

Age 5 to Puberty

As your child matures, you will be able to start passing on more and more responsibility for details of self-care. From this time, you will be able to use diabetes classes, support groups, and camps to supplement your roles in education and emotional support. Use *Living Well* as a source book for answering questions and offering guidance. You and your doctor will form a team determining regimen choices for the child to consider. You will work together to build the positive motivation needed for following the resulting team program.

Teenage years

At this time, the basic approach of *Living Well* may be the most effective way of bypassing or quieting rebellion against diabetic regimen. See your child as capable of making responsible choices, as needing to participate fully in decisions about his or her health and life-style, and as the final authority over what he or she actually does with his or her life. With this point of view, there is a basis for negotiation that cannot exist if you hold onto this responsibility and authority. You are also more likely to keep communication open about what is going on with diabetes in your teen's life. Children who learn well from written material may be able to start working directly with *Living Well*, although you may need to help. (This book is written at the high school level.)

CHOOSING THE LEVEL OF REGIMEN

For all but the very young, your doctor, your child, and you must work together to find a level of diabetic regimen and control that will work for all parties. Often the physician advises against the intensive regimen because of the greater dangers of insulin reactions in childhood. Children are usually much more active and engage in their activities with such intensity that the onset of reactions may be difficult to notice. Often they wish not to appear different because of their diabetes, and they may want to hide their vulnerability. The level of awareness demanded by the intensive regimen might cause some children to become preoccupied with their illness and some parents to become obsessive about it.

On the other hand, with the right combination of child, parents, and doctor, many children have learned to manage diabetes very carefully and live full, exuberant lives. The decision about the level of regimen a child is to learn to follow must be reached through thoughtful discussion between the whole family and the physician. The factors you will need to balance include

1. The likely long-term value of avoiding chronic high blood sugar levels.

2. The need to avoid frequent insulin reactions.

3. The feelings of your child and yourself.

4. Your child's age and learning skills.

5. Your child's growth pattern and overall health (chronically high blood sugar can slow growth and the onset of puberty).

DIABETIC COMPLICATIONS

Diabetes carries with it the risk of secondary disorders that may develop later in your child's life. No subject in parenting requires more sensitivity than these possible complications. Along with insulin reactions and diabetic coma, they constitute a major threat and source of fear for parents and children alike. When your child begins to be aware of diabetic complications, you will need to convey carefully the nature of the threat and tell your child what to do to reduce the risk. (Your child may come to you in distress after hearing a diabetic relative or friend of the family who has developed serious complications.) There are several important points to make:

• Some diabetics develop a complication, but many do not. The authors of *Living Well*, after 170 years of diabetes altogether, all see clearly, have no kidney disease, and have only minor complications.

• Diabetics can do many things to lessen their risk of developing complications.

• Treatment for diabetic complications is improving; in many cases, treatment enables the person with diabetes to avoid disabilities altogether.

- If your child is old enough, discuss the concept of risk, and how everyone is at risk and has to learn to deal with the fears this produces. Life has threats, but we live well by remembering life's promises more than the threats.

- In general, answer the questions your child brings up, but don't flood him or her with too much information. Keep a balance between the facts and the emotional reassurance you offer.

You should not force information about complications on your child, and, above all, you should never use threats of dire consequences to encourage your child to follow regimen. Either practice is likely to build more anxiety than adherence. Carefully inspect any booklets or audiovisual presentations on complications before using them. Old educational materials often use frightening, worst-case photos and threatening language. Even current publications on complications are seldom written with sensitivity to the emotional needs of the reader.

Before discussing complications with your child, read Chapter 15 and the sections on preventive measures in Chapter 17. Deal with your own feelings about these threats first, so you can be calm in helping your child.

DIABETES POWER STRUGGLES

Any parents and children may develop power struggles over the children's behavior. With diabetes, however, these conflicts can take on an extreme level of emotion when "not doing the right thing" appears to threaten the child's very survival. As the parent, you may feel anxious, frantic, and possibly angry when your child "forgets" insulin repeatedly or eats excessive amounts of sweets. If your anxiety causes you to try to force your child to follow regimen, you may simply incite your child to rebel even more.

You can do several things to avoid turning a matter of such genuine concern into a full power struggle:

- Deal with your own feelings apart from the situation. Don't dump them on your child.

- Ask your child to help you understand what is happening and what changes are needed to handle the problem. Work with your child rather than giving commands.

- Look at your child's behavior in terms of what is happening in his or her life. How does having diabetes function to reward the child with attention; to allow him or her to escape obligations or responsibilities; or to express feelings he or she can't express directly? How can you help satisfy these needs directly?

- Set goals together, with a clear understanding of how you will both know when they are met. If it fits your style of parenting, set appropriate rewards and penalties.

- Work with the basic understanding that you have a problem to solve together, not that your child is the problem.

Finally, understand that in some matters of regimen there is room for a few little vacations. Sweets, for instance, are not poison to a diabetic; they are simply something to be eaten with great moderation. Don't let your child think that the only time he or she can eat a dessert or piece of candy is during an insulin reaction. Dietitians have found that regular nondietetic ice cream at mealtime does not increase blood sugar level seriously, so long as it is not covered with gooey toppings.

DIABETIC FOR A DAY

Parents and diabetes professionals have gained remarkable empathy by living as diabetics for a day or more. They test their blood several times a day, take injections of sterile water, watch their diet, and follow an exercise program. If you care to enter into your child's reality in this way, you will discover a new level of respect for what he or she must do each day. And your youngster will be delighted that you have taken this dramatic step to see the world in this new way.

The theme of empathy this simulation teaches is the foundation for good parenting. When your love for your child is supported by this sort of respect and understanding, you both find that you can live well with diabetes.

BOOKS FOR PARENTS OF A DIABETIC YOUTH

Diabetes. Lee Ducat and Sherry Suib Cohen. Harper and Row (1983). A complete guide to healthier living for parents, children, and young adults who have insulin-dependent diabetes.

368

The first author of this book, Lee Ducat, is the founder of the Juvenile Diabetes Foundation and the mother of a diabetic. She has drawn on her own experience as well as that of the patients, families, and doctors involved in JDF. The book is written as a "coping manual, a practical guide," with tips to help young diabetics and their families live well with diabetes.

It includes information on "how to deal with doctors, teachers, babysitters, and other children; how to set and achieve reasonable goals for testing, diet and exercise; how to handle camp, birthday parties, school, sports and travel; what to do in emergencies; advice on dating, sex, marriage and pregnancy; and how to deal with the anger and depression this disease can cause." This valuable resource has chapters on the needs of diabetic babies, youngsters, teenagers, and young adults.

You can order a copy by calling 1-800-242-7737.

Whole Parent / Whole Child, A Parent's Guide to Raising Children with a Chronic Health Condition. Broatch Haig and Patricia Moynihan. DCI/CHRONIMED Publishing, Minneapolis, Minnesota (1989).

While covering a broader range of conditions than diabetes, the authors (a dietitian and a nurse specialist) are diabetes educators. Their book is based on years of helping parents and children deal with the demands of diabetes.

This book can be ordered by calling CHRONIMED's toll free number, 1-800-848-2793. Ask for a catalog of other publications on diabetes.

What Does It Feel Like to Have Diabetes? Denise J. Bradley. Charles C. Thomas, Springfield, Illinois.

This autobiographical book was written by a 27-year-old woman who has had diabetes since the age of 3.

The American Diabetes Association has a number of publications in its catalog, including *Especially for Parents*, a package of articles reprinted from *Diabetes Forecast* newsletter, cookbooks, pamphlets, and the following two books. You can order all of these and request the catalog by calling the ADA's toll free order number, 1-800-ADA-DISC.

Children with Diabetes. Linda M. Siminerio and Jean Betschart. For parents, teachers, and others who work with diabetic children.

This book covers all the details of diabetic management, takes a sensitive look at children's psychological needs, and offers suggestions for promoting a positive and supportive home environment. Order from the American Diabetes Association.

Kid's Corner. For children with diabetes. Children aged 8 to 12 have fun as they learn about diabetes through this booklet of puzzles and games. Order from the American Diabetes Association.

A Book on Diabetes for Brothers and Sisters. Linda Siminerio. Children's Hospital of Pittsburgh, Pennsylvania.

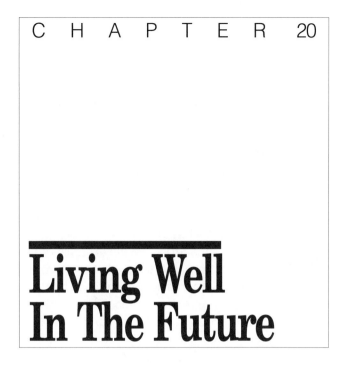

C H A P T E R 20

Living Well In The Future

INTRODUCTION

The pace of diabetes research continues to accelerate. As researchers march toward a "cure," what will this mean for those of us with diabetes? First, it will become easier and easier to control our blood sugar, either through new technological devices or advances in pancreas and islet cell transplants. Second, new ways to prevent or treat complications will be discovered. Third, researchers are investigating the feasibility of actually preventing the development of diabetes in those at risk. Intimately tied to each of these areas will be a better understanding of the immune reactions that cause diabetes, as well as the genes that predispose or prevent the development of diabetes and its complications.

EASIER BLOOD SUGAR CONTROL

External insulin pumps worn outside the body have been available for several years. However, implantable pumps (about the size of a hockey puck but likely to become smaller) surgically inserted under the skin are in the final phases of experimental trials. The pump is filled

371

approximately monthly by injecting very concentrated insulin into a reservoir in the pump, which then releases insulin as programmed by a hand-held remote control device. However, the user must still test blood sugars frequently—and this means pricking the finger each time. On the horizon are two advances which will alleviate this concern: the noninvasive glucose meter and the implantable glucose sensor.

Several companies and researchers are developing meters that can read sugar levels within the body without drawing even a drop of blood! One device measures the absorbance of laser or near infra-red (NIR) light beams directed through the skin in blood vessels of the finger or wrist. Another directs the laser beam into the watery fluid near the front of the eye (the aqueous humor) and calculates the sugar based on the deflection of the beam caused by the sugar concentration. We expect that meters using these technologies or some variation will proceed through their trial periods, become approved by the FDA, and will be marketed to health professionals and the public—but at a cost (at least initially) probably 10 to 50 times the cost of invasive meters!

Work is also proceeding to develop an implantable glucose sensor. In the past, development has been plagued by technical problems: The sensor clogs or accuracy fails in a few months. It is likely that the technical problems will be solved in the next few years, and the implantable sensor, in conjunction with the implantable pump, will create a true artificial pancreas.

In the meantime, progress is being made in the development of aerosolized insulin, either through a nasal spray or inhaled through the mouth, similar to the familiar inhalers for asthma. The oral inhalers appear to be less irritating than the nasal spray, and are absorbed more efficiently into the lungs and bloodstream. Lastly, and surprisingly, we have heard about a pill that supposedly has been shown to deliver insulin into the bloodstream! We have been unable to learn more about these preliminary studies, which were carried out at the Hadassah-Hebrew University Medical Center in Jerusalem.

As for the traditional insulin preparations, we expect that in the next few years, all the animal-source insulins will be replaced by synthetic genetically engineered insulin. These are pure and not dependent on an external supply of animal pancreases. However, we hope the manufacturers keep working to genetically engineer a variety of activity profiles (onset, peak, and duration) to add flexibility to the user's armamentarium. In particular, we would like to see some tinkering to develop a human Ultralente insulin that matches the longer duration of the existing beef/pork Ultralente (see Ultralente anecdote in Chapter 5).

Some new drugs on the horizon (all experimental) may prove helpful in blood sugar regulation, particularly in type II (noninsulin dependent) diabetes. First, a chromium supplement (in the form of a pill, chromium picolinate) has been shown not only to decrease blood lipids (total cholesterol and LDL) by about 10 percent but also blood glucose by about 25 percent. It was particularly effective in American Indians, who have a high incidence of noninsulin-dependent diabetes. A second drug, insulinotropin, is actually a naturally occurring hormone produced in the intestines when we eat. It stimulates release of insulin from the pancreas, but its insulin-releasing effect diminishes as blood sugar falls (a desirable characteristic). Thus, it may be a useful substitute for insulin in those type II patients who need insulin. Lastly, a drug called amylin, naturally produced in the beta-cells of the pancreas along with insulin, may also help to avoid hypoglycemia in type I diabetes. Insulinotropin and amylin both must be injected.

Progress has also been significant on the transplant front. First, survival of patients following pancreas transplantation has continued to improve, and their new pancreases are producing insulin for longer periods of time. Second, islet cell transplantation researchers are exploring ways to prevent the recipient's rejection of the foreign tissue. Various materials are being tested to coat or encapsulate the islet cells, preventing the cells from being attacked but allowing insulin and glucose to pass through.

An alternative approach uses targeted antibodies (genetically engineered monoclonal antibodies) to prevent the patient's own immune mechanisms from destroying the transplanted cells. Another method has been used in rats to fool the body into believing that the transplanted cells were its own. The islet cells were transplanted into a gland in the neck called the thymus. Soon the procedure will be tested in humans.

A limitation of the above methods has been the availability of sufficient tissue, either pancreas or islet cells, to treat all those who may benefit. A new method, using genetic engineering and a line of cells that can be grown in a test tube (hence suitable for large-scale production), may produce an artificial beta-cell. It uses mouse pituitary cells that have been engineered to produce insulin and respond to glucose. However, additional work needs to be done to remove some of the "bugs" (e.g., cells start releasing insulin before blood sugar is high enough and also secrete a mouse hormone that may affect humans). It will likely be three to five years before human trials. The prospects are good that one or more of these transplant approaches will soon be successful.

PREVENTION AND TREATMENT OF COMPLICATIONS

We believe the next decade will see considerable research in the genetics of both type I and type II diabetes mellitus. One particularly exciting area will be the detection and study of those genes that either predispose to the development of complications, or protect against their development. As we discussed in earlier chapters, some of us in optimal control of our diabetes will develop complications, and others in poor control will manage to avoid most if not all complications. Our own genetic makeups will likely explain some of this variability. For example, a recent study suggested that a particular kind of diabetic neuropathy (cardiovascular autonomic neuropathy) was strongly associated with a particular genetic marker. The Diabetes Control and Complications Trial (see Chapter 17) may provide an excellent pool of patients to study genetically for this purpose, since data on their level of control and their development of complications will already have been collected.

Several drugs are being developed and tested that hold the promise of preventing or treating complications. Some of these were mentioned in Chapter 17, like ACE inhibitors for preventing nephropathy, and sorbinil for treating neuropathy. Much more study needs to be done. Since many diabetic complications involve abnormalities of the blood vessels, particularly the new growth of abnormal vessels as in retinopathy, trials of drugs that retard vessel growth (angiogenesis inhibitors) are being considered for people with diabetes. One example is alpha-interferon, which has been used in the treatment of leukemia and AIDS. However, the potential benefits must be weighed against cost and side effects, particularly where a generally satisfactory therapy (laser photocoagulation) already exists.

PREVENTING THE DEVELOPMENT OF DIABETES

Researchers know that type I diabetes is an autoimmune disease—where the person's own antibodies attack the insulin-producing beta cells of the pancreas. Only recently have researchers been able to determine those who are the most likely to develop diabetes *before* most of their beta cells have been destroyed (a slow process) and before they have developed typical clinical symptoms. Now large-scale studies are beginning to screen close relatives of those with diabetes for level of antibodies that predict a high risk of developing diabetes in the future. Those individuals with a high likelihood of developing diabetes will be offered the opportunity to participate in clinical trials to determine if the diabetes can be prevented. Drugs such as nicotinamide or immunosuppressives like cyclosporine or azathioprine (Imuran) may be used. All of these drugs have significant side-effects, however, and the potential benefits must be weighed against the risks.

Research is also beginning on a large scale to identify the genes responsible for both type I and type II diabetes. Just as the cloning and sequencing of the gene responsible for cystic fibrosis have stimulated further research into the cause and cure for cystic fibrosis, so too will genetic research into diabetes help advance treatment for people with diabetes. The National Institutes of Health and the American Diabetes Association (assisted by grants from private industry) are beginning major projects to develop family trees and establish banks of cells from family members that can be studied by a wide range of collaborating researchers, all hoping to identify the many different genes involved and their complex interplay.

To conclude, we believe that there is a very good chance that some form of "cure" will be a reality by the year 2000. The future prospects are truly exciting for those of us with diabetes.

A Diabetes
Survival Kit

Living well with diabetes begins with staying alive. So this positive book on self-care highlights three potential threats diabetes presents and the things you can do to tame them. Being knowledgeable about these subjects is of the highest priority in your diabetes management.

1. *Insulin reactions.* Low blood sugar (hypoglycemia) can lead to confusion and unconsciousness. You need to know what causes very low blood sugar, the symptoms that you experience, and the treatment. Chapter 8 provides the details of insulin reactions and how to deal with them.

2. *Diabetic coma.* You also need to learn the causes and symtoms of diabetic ketoacidosis and coma, which can result from very high blood sugar (hyperglycemia), omitted insulin shots, poorly managed illness or infections, or extreme stress. The Diabetic Ketoacidosis and Sick Day Management sections that follow discuss diabetic coma.

3. *Handling infections.* Small infections can become severe, and severe ones can lead to the diabetic coma. The section on ketoacidosis

and Sick Day Management, and the foot-care section of Chapter 17 are good sources of information on handling infections.

These three threats require that you

- Never omit an insulin injection unless your doctor okays it.

- Always carry candy, sugar, or glucose tablets with you to treat reactions.

- Always wear a diabetes identification bracelet or necklace.

- Treat all wounds, scratches, and punctures to prevent infections.

Report illness or infections to your doctor, especially when they increase blood sugar levels or when you have ketones in your urine. See your doctor without delay if you need treatment.

Diabetic Ketoacidosis and Sick Day Management

Diabetic ketoacidosis—or ketosis—is a condition of type I, insulin-dependent, diabetes in which blood glucose and ketones rise to high levels. This state can be dangerous for a person with diabetes, leading to diabetic coma if not treated. It usually responds to prompt treatment, however, so you should know the symptoms and steps you can take when the symptoms occur.

Causes

    The physical stress of illness or infected wounds

    Great emotional stress

    Chronically high blood sugar levels combined with stress

    Omitted insulin

    Any combination of the above

Initial Signs and Symptoms

    Positive urine ketone and glucose tests

    High blood sugar tests (above 240 mg/dl)

    Dehydration, thirst, dry mouth

    Excessive, frequent urination

Nausea, vomiting, abdominal pain

Fatigue or weakness

Fever

Blurred vision

Signs and Symptoms as Condition Advances Toward Diabetic Coma

Flushed, dry skin

Fruity odor on breath

Sunken eyes

Deep, labored breathing

Pulse usually rapid

Unconsciousness

You may need to be treated in the hospital if your condition advances toward diabetic coma or does not respond to home treatment. Stay in touch with your doctor from the very first signs of ketosis.

(Note that insulin reactions, which can also lead to unconsciousness, are marked by much more rapid onset than ketosis, shallow breathing, normal-smelling breath, and low blood sugar.)

Treatment of Ketoacidosis

Any level of ketosis marked by a positive test for ketones in your urine needs your immediate attention. (People with kidney disease, especially, should be aware of the symptoms and begin treatment immediately when urine tests show ketones.)

Test urine and blood frequently: When you are ill—especially when you are vomiting, have diarrhea, or are feverish—you should test your urine for ketones and test your blood glucose. Infected wounds also can produce ketosis. Test every two or three hours until the results are normal.

Confer with your doctor: When you are ill and have ketones in your urine, ask your doctor for guidance in handling the situation. Your doctor will usually suggest extra shots of regular insulin to bring blood glucose and ketone levels down. The amount of insulin needed will be determined according to your body weight, blood sugar level, and severity of illness.

(After you have dealt with this level of illness a few times, your doctor may tell you that you know enough to handle it with minimal medical guidance. But any time you do not see improvement within six or eight hours, ask for your doctor's help.)

Continue taking insulin: You should never omit insulin, even when you are ill and unable to eat solid food. The stress of illness itself raises blood sugar levels.

Continue eating: You need to continue eating and drinking foods and fluids with caloric value, even if your blood sugar is high and you are vomiting or have diarrhea.

Take in at least 10 to 20 grams of carbohydrate every one to two hours. Possible sources include: 1/3 cup flavored gelatin, 1/2 cup vanilla ice cream, 1/2 cup custard, 1/2 cup orange juice, 3/4 cup ginger ale (not diet), 1/2 cup regular cola, or 1 cup Gatorade.

If you have trouble keeping food down, take smaller quantities every fifteen to thirty minutes.

Limit activity: Even if you feel able to exercise, when you have high blood sugar and ketones in your urine, *don't*. Exercising at this time actually raises blood sugar.

A P P E N D I X

Resources for Living Well

DIABETES IDENTIFICATION

You should wear, at all times, a bracelet or necklace identifying you as having diabetes and giving a number to call for information in case of emergency. The following services maintain 24-hour hotlines, where details of your diabetes care are available to medical personnel from anywhere in the world. Medic Alert says, "This identification could save your life. Any diabetic who has passed out from insulin shock or coma will agree.

Medic Alert Foundation International
P.O. Box 1009
Turlock, CA 95381
(800) 432-5378
(209) 668-3333
Medic Alert Foundation provides attractive I.D. bracelets and necklaces and has a toll-free number with medical information.

Med-Fax
618 Venice Blvd.
Marina del Rey, CA 90291
(213) 821-1984
Med-Fax is a highly specialized emergency data system that allows one to store emergency medical information in the MED-FAX Voice Computer. In an emergency, the computer speaks your medical file directly over the telephone to physicians or trauma centers worldwide.

ORGANIZATIONS AND SOURCES OF INFORMATION

American Diabetes Association
1660 Duke Street
Alexandria, VA 22314
Or call 1-800-ADA-DISC
The American Diabetes Association (ADA) supports research, education, and public awareness programs relating to both insulin-dependent and noninsulin-dependent diabetes. A membership fee of $20 a year provides monthly issues of *Diabetes Forecast* and automatic membership in a local chapter.

Juvenile Diabetes Foundation International
432 Park Ave. So.
New York 10016
(800)223-1138
The Juvenile Diabetes Foundation (JDF) is a volunteer organization specializing in insulin-dependent diabetes. It has a network of chapters worldwide and raises funds for diabetes research. Chapters provide helpful brochures as well as personal contact. A quarterly newsletter is published for JDF members.

National Diabetes Information Clearinghouse
Box NDIC, 9000 Rockville Pike
Bethesda, MD 20892
(301) 468-2162
The National Diabetes Information Clearinghouse (NDIC) works to increase knowledge and understanding about diabetes among patients, health professionals, and the public. It provides responses to inquiries, and resources for patient education, including publications, professional and patient education programs, and an online data base. Call or write to request NDIC's publications list. Diabetes Dateline is the organization's newsletter.

American Association of Diabetes Educators

500 North Michigan Ave., #1400

Chicago, IL 60611

The American Association of Diabetes Educators (AADE) publishes a directory of diabetes education programs. Write to them for more information.

Joslin Diabetes Foundation, Inc., Publications Department

One Joslin Plaza

Boston, MA 02215

Joslin Clinic was the pioneer treatment center for diabetes care. The Foundation provides information and literature concerning diabetes.

HCF Diabetes Foundation

P.O. Box 22124

Lexington, KY 40522

The HCF Diabetes Foundation publishes *Diabetes and Nutrition* ($6 per year), a newsletter based on the work of James W. Anderson, M.D., concerning the healthful benefits of high-carbohydrate, high-fiber diets. Other publications are available.

International Diabetes Center (IDC)

5000 West 39th Street

Minneapolis, MN 55416

(612) 927-3393

The goal of this organization is to help persons with diabetes have fulfilling and active lifestyles. IDC publishes books, pamphlets, and Living Well With Diabetes, a quarterly magazine. All publications are distributed through CHRONIMED Publishing. For a catalog call, 1-800-848-2793.

Sugarfree Center

P.O. Box 114

Van Nuys, CA 91408

1-800-972-2323

Provides general diabetes information. (Also see listing under Diabetic Supplies.)

Other sources of information include companies that produce diabetic supplies. You may request specific booklets and catalogs of publications from the following:

Ames Division, Miles Laboratories, Inc.
P.O. Box 70, Elkhart, IN 46515

Becton-Dickinson
Rochelle Park, NJ 07662

Eli Lilly & Co.
Indianapolis, IN 46285

Monoject Division
Sherwood Medical
St. Louis, MO 63166

Pfizer Laboratories
New York, NY

Squibb-Novo
120 Alexander St.
Princeton, NJ 08540

DIABETES MAGAZINES

American Diabetes Association
General Membership
P.O. Box 2055
Harlan, IA 51593-0238

Diabetes Forecast is the most complete magazine for people with diabetes. Published by the American Diabetes Association, it includes reports on new research, personal stories, practical tips on diabetes care, and articles for children. Membership is $20 per year. Reprints and special topic packages are available.

Center for Diabetes Education
Ames Division
Miles Laboratories, Inc.
P.O. Box 70
Elkhart, IN 46515

Diabetes in the News is a magazine featuring diabetes management and lifestyle articles. It is published every other month by the Ames Center for Diabetes Education. Subscriptions are $9 per year.

CHRONIMED Publishing Inc. (formerly DCI Publishing)

P.O. Box 739
Wayzata, MN 55391

Living Well With Diabetes is a quarterly magazine produced in coopera-
tion with the International Diabetes Center. The magazine includes
informative articles on self-care and current research, as well as the
catalog for discount supplies from CHRONIMED Pharmacy. You can
order a free two-issue trial subscription by calling 1-800-848-0614.
Subscription fee is $6.

Diabetes Self Management

P.O. Box 52890
Boulder, CO 80322-2890

Diabetes Self-Management is a bimonthly magazine containing practical self-care articles. Subscription is $36 per year.

SOME BOOKS ON DIABETES

The following books are available from CHRONIMED Publishing:

Learning to Live Well With Diabetes, by Donnell D. Etzwiler and others
from the International Diabetes Center. This up-to-date, comprehensive and easy-to-understand manual helps people with diabetes work
with their diabetes team to improve control and quality of life.

The Physician Within—Taking Charge of Your Well Being, by Catherine
Feste. This book is about self-motivation for people who are trying to
follow either a pattern of healthy living or a specific medical regimen.

Exchanges for All Occasions—Meeting the Challenge of Diabetes, by
Marion J. Franz. This book helps everyone use the exchange system for
meal planning in almost any situation.

CHRONIMED Publishing also has pamphlets from the International
Diabetes Center available through their catalog. Request a catalog from
CHRONIMED Publishing, P.O. Box 47945, Minneapolis, MN 55391,
or call 1-800-848-2793.

Other books available in bookstores or libraries:

Diabetes, by Lee Ducat and Sherry Suib Cohen. A complete guide to healthier living for parents, children, and young adults who have insulin-dependent diabetes. Harper and Row (1983). You can order a copy by calling 1-800-242-7737.

Diabetic Child and Young Adult, by Mimi Belmonte (1983).

Diabetes: A Practical Guide To Healthy Living, by James W. Anderson. Arco, Inc., publishes this guide for general diabetes management written by Dr. Anderson, with a special section on the HCF diet plan. Warner Books (1983). Order from HCF Diabetes Foundation, P.O. Box 22124, Lexington, KY 40522.

The American Diabetes Association publishes a large number of books, pamphlets, and reprints of articles from Diabetes Forecast. Below are some of the ADA titles available.

Family Cookbook—Volumes 1, 2, and 3.

Kid's Corner, ADA (1983). Children have fun as they learn about diabetes through this booklet of puzzles and games. For children ages 8 through 12 with diabetes.

Children with Diabetes, by Linda M. Siminerio and Jean Betschart. ADA (1986). For parents, teachers, and others who work with diabetic children. It covers all the details of diabetic management, takes a sensitive look at children's psychological needs, and offers suggestions for promoting a positive and supportive home environment.

Diabetes in the Family, ADA (1987). This book deals with day-to-day issues of diet and self-care as well as lifetime issues such as employment and marriage.

Diabetes: Reach for Health and Freedom, by Dorothea Sims. ADA (1984). Learn how a person with diabetes not only survives but excels. For both patients and professionals.

Diabetes A to Z, ADA (1988). An expanded and updated version of the former *Guide to Good Living.* Arranged in dictionary format for easy reference, this book covers the medical concerns of a person with diabetes, as well as some less conventional topics, such as tax tips, dealing with Halloween and Valentine's Day, dancing, driving, and handling feelings of loneliness.

The ADA publications listed can be ordered from:

American Diabetes Association
National Service Center
1660 Duke Street
Alexandria, VA 22314
Or call 1-800-ADA-DISC

Diabetes: Caring for Your Emotions As Well As Your Health, by Jerry Edelwich and Archie Brodsky (1986).

The Diabetic's Book: All Your Questions Answered, by June Biermann and Barbara Toohey. Tarcher, Santa Monica, CA (1981).

The Diabetic's Total Health Book, by June Biermann and Barbara Toohey. Tarcher, Santa Monica, CA (1988).

The Peripatetic Diabetic, by June Biermann and Barbara Toohey. Tarcher, Santa Monica, CA (1984).

The Diabetic Woman, by June Biermann, Barbara Toohey, and Dr. Lois Jovanovic. Tarcher, Santa Monica, CA (1987).

FILMS AND AUDIOVISUALS

Films, videos, and audiotapes are available on different aspects of diabetes care. Your library, local chapter of ADA, or your diabetes educator or doctor may have these resources. Some of the titles available are:

Diabetes: Focus on Feelings
The Sugar Film
Gestational Diabetes—Great Expectations
Know Your Diabetes: Know Yourself

DISCOUNT DIABETES SUPPLIES

The following companies advertise in the ADA's *Diabetes Forecast* magazine. They all have toll-free numbers, so calling to check on prices is free to the caller. Also inquire about any specials they may be offering.

CHRONIMED Pharmacy
P.O. Box 47945
Minneapolis, MN 55391
1-800-848-2793

Diabetic Express
P.O. Box 80037
Canton, OH 44708
1-800-338-4656

Diabetic Information Services, Inc.
5726 Cortez Rd., #149
Bradenton, FL 34210
1-800-633-7167

Diabetic Promotions
P.O. Box 5400
Willowick, OH 44095-0400
1-800-433-1477
(216) 934-6185

Diabetic Resource Centers
8181 N. Stadium Dr.
Houston, TX 77054
1-800-622-5587
(713)797-1726

H-S Medical Supplies
P.O. Box 42
Whitehall, PA 18052
1-800-344-7633

Hospital Center Pharmacy
433 Brookline Ave.
Boston MA 02215
1-800-824-2401

Insur-Aid Diabetic Supplies
P.O. Box 8955
Roanoke, VA 24014
1-800-944-8141

Jocelyn Bischoff's Diabetic
2200 Airport Blvd.
Freedom, CA 95019
1-800-537-0404

National Diabetic Pharmacies
P.O. Box 7587
Roanoke, VA 24019
1-800-467-8546

Self Care, Inc.
1289 21st Ave.
San Francisco, CA 94122
1-800-654-9801
415-664-1100

Sugar Free Center
P.O. Box 114
Van Nuys, CA 91408
1-800-972-2323

Sugar Happy Diabetes Supplies
3715 Balboa St.
San Francisco, CA 94121
1-800-347-4848
415-347-4737

Thriftee Home Diabetes Center
1426 E. Fletcher Ave.,
Tampa, FL 32612
1-800-258-9559

INDEX

389

CHRONIMED PUBLISHING
BOOKS OF RELATED INTEREST

When Diabetes Complicates Your Life by Joseph Juliano, M.D. Dr. Juliano, an endocrinologist and research scientist, has had diabetes for 29 years and is now totally blind. He knows firsthand what it's like to combat the effects of diabetes. Empowering readers to find the motivation and information to control diabetes, Dr. Juliano shows how to avoid complications and overcome them if they occur.
004207   ISBN 1-56561-012-1 $9.95

Diabetes: A Guide to Living Well by Ernest Lowe and Gary Arsham, M.D., Ph.D. This comprehensive and up-to-date guide helps the person with diabetes design a program of individualized self-care and gain the willingness to follow it. It also tells how to deal with diet, exercise, stress, emotions, negative beliefs, and self-image.
004208   ISBN 1-56561-009-1 $12.95

It's Time to Learn about Diabetes by Jean Betschart, M.N., R.N., C.D.E. From fun exercises to family vacations, *It's Time to Learn About Diabetes* has everything school-age kids need to know about diabetes. It's a delightful, entertaining, and easy-to-use workbook that not only teaches children about what's happening to their bodies, but also helps them take care of themselves. Jean Betschart is president of the American Association of Diabetes Educators and coauthor of *Children with Diabetes*.
004084   ISBN 0-937721-80-8 $9.95

A Touch of Diabetes by Lois Jovanovic-Peterson, M.D., Charles M. Peterson, M.D., and Morton Stone. Everything people with newly diagnosed noninsulin-dependent diabetes need to know, from curbing potential complications to counting calories, is in this authoritative and easy-to understand guide. Written by two of the foremost authorities on diabetes–Dr. Lois Jovanovic-Peterson and Dr. Charles M. Peterson–and the editor of *Diabetes in the News* magazine, Morton Stone, this book clearly shows how to control diabetes and improve quality of life.
004092   ISBN 0-937721-89-1 $7.95

When a Family gets Diabetes by Marge Heegaard, M.A., A.T.R., and Chris Ternand, M.D. This unique book uses art therapy to help children with diabetes and their families understand and verbally express their feelings about diabetes, themselves, and others. Here they draw pictures that relate to certain aspects of diabetes and discuss why they drew what they did.
004067   ISBN 0-937721-75-1 $6.95

Diabetes 101: A Pure and Simple Guide for People who Use Insulin by Richard O. Dolinar, M.D., and Betty Page Brackenridge, M.S., R.D., C.D.E. Here's a clear and easy-to-understand guide to the basic information needed by people using insulin to control diabetes, especially those newly diagnosed.
004065   ISBN 0-937721-63-8 $7.95

Diabetes Care Made Easy by Allison Nemaniec, R.N., Gretchen Kauth, R.D., and Marion Franz, R.D., M.S. Illustrated by Jan Westberg. Written and designed for both children and adults with limited reading skills, this breezy and easy-to-read book explains how to exercise and eat for better health, prevent foot problems, test blood sugar, cope with emotions, take insulin, and more.
004210   ISBN 1-56561-013-X $9.95

Diabetes: Actively Staying Healthy by Marion Franz, M.S., R.D., C.D.E., and Jane Norstrom, M.A. This is an essential and complete reference guide for diabetes and exercise. Highly motivational and with the latest facts, it has everything you need to know to participate safely at all levels of physical activity.
004056   ISBN 0-937721-57-3 $9.95

Learning to Live Well With Diabetes by Marion Franz, R.D., M.S., C.D.E., Donnell D. Etzwiler, M.D., Judy Ostrom Joynes, M.A., R.M., C.D.E., and Priscilla M. Hollander, M.D., Ph.D. You won't find a more comprehensive, authoritative, and easy-to-understand guide on managing diabetes than *Learning to Live Well With Diabetes*. Written by more than 25 prominent diabetes experts, this revised and updated edition reflects the latest medical advances, technologies, and research. In straightforward language, it explains how to take charge of your diabetes and live an active, healthy life. Plus, it contains over 200 useful illustrations, charts, and tables.
004083   ISBN 0-937721-79-4 $24.95

Managing Type II Diabetes by Arlene Monk, R.D., C.D.E., et al. Here's a basic guide for those who want to control Type II, or noninsulin-dependent, diabetes–rather than have it control them. Written by a team of diabetes specialists, this down-to-earth manual clearly explains what Type II diabetes is and how to manage it.
004022   ISBN 0-937721-24-7 $9.95

The Physician Within by Catherine Feste. Here internationally renowned health motivation specialist, Cathy Feste, focuses on motivating those with a health challenge, and anyone else, to stay on their regimen and follow healthy behavior.
004019   ISBN 0-937721-19-0 $8.95

Let Them Eat Cake by Virginia N. White with Rosa A. Mo., R.D. If you're looking for delicious and healthy pies, cookies, puddings, and cakes, this book will give you your just desserts. With easy, step-by-step instructions, this innovative cookbook features complete nutrition information, the latest exchange values, and tips on making your favorite snacks more healthful.
004206   ISBN 1-56561-011-3 $12.95

All-American Low-Fat Meals in Minutes by M.J. Smith R.D., L.D., M.A. Filled with tantalizing recipes and valuable tips, this cookbook makes great-tasting low-fat foods a snap for holidays, special occasions, or everyday. Most recipes take only minutes to prepare.
004079   ISBN 0-937721-73-5 $12.95

Convenience Food Facts by Marion Franz, R.D., M.S. and Arlene Monk, R.D., C.D.E. Includes complete nutrition information, tips, and exchange values on more than 1,500 popular name-brand processed foods commonly found in grocery store freezers and shelves. Helps you plan easy-to-prepare, nutritious meals.
004081   ISBN 0-937721-77-8 $10.95

Fast Food Facts by Marion Franz, R.D., M.S. This revised and up-to-date best-seller shows how to make smart nutrition choices at fast food restaurants–and tells what to avoid. Includes complete nutrition information on more than 1,000 menu offerings from the 21 largest fast food chains.
Standard-size edition   004068   ISBN 0-937721-67-0 $6.95
Pocket edition   004073   ISBN 0-937721-69-7 $4.95

Exchanges for All Occasions by Marion Franz, R.D., M.S. Exchanges and meal planning suggestions for just about any occasion, sample meal plans, special tips for people with diabetes, and more.
004201   ISBN 1-56561-005-9 $12.95

Buy them at your local bookstore
or use this convenient coupon for ordering.

Order by mail:

**C H R O N I M E D
PHARMACY**
P.O. Box 47945
Minneapolis, MN 55447-9727

Or order by phone:

1-800-848-2793
1-800-444-5951 *(non-metro area of Minnesota)*
612-546-1146 *(Minneapolis/St. Paul metro area)*
Please have your credit card number ready.

Please send me the books I have checked above. I am enclosing $. (Please add $3.00 to this order to cover postage and handling. Minnesota residents add 6.5% sales tax.) Send check or money order, no cash or C.O.D.'s. Prices are subject to change without notice.

Name _____

Address _____

City _____ State _____ Zip _____

Allow 4 to 6 weeks for delivery.
Quantity discounts available upon request.